THE NATURE OF CITIES

Studies in Comparative History

Essays from the

Shelby Cullom Davis Center for Historical Studies

Animals in Human Histories: The Mirror of Nature and Culture
Edited by Mary J. Henninger-Voss

The Animal/Human Boundary: Historical Perspectives
Edited by Angela N. H. Creager and William Chester Jordan

Conversion: Old Worlds and New
Edited by Kenneth Mills and Anthony Grafton

Conversion in Late Antiquity and the Early Middle Ages: Seeing and Believing
Edited by Kenneth Mills and Anthony Grafton

Corrupt Histories
Edited by Emmanuel Kreike and William Chester Jordan

Repositioning Migration History: New Directions in Modern Continental Migration, Citizenship, and Community
Edited by Marc S. Rodriquez

The Nature of Cities: Culture, Landscape, and Urban Space
Edited by Andrew C. Isenberg

A Publication of the Shelby Cullom Davis Center for Historical Studies
Princeton University

Directors

Lawrence Stone (1974–1988)
Natalie Zemon Davis (1988–1994)
William Chester Jordan (1994–1999)
Anthony T. Grafton (1999–2003)
Gyan Prakash (2003–)

THE NATURE OF CITIES

Edited by

Andrew C. Isenberg

University of Rochester Press

First published 2005
Transferred to digital printing 2016

University of Rochester Press
668 Mt. Hope Avenue, Rochester, NY 14620, USA
www.urpress.com
and Boydell & Brewer Limited
PO Box 9, Woodbridge, Suffolk IP12 3DF, UK
www.boydellandbrewer.com

ISSN: 1539-4905
ISBN: 978-1-58046-220-4

Library of Congress Cataloging-in-Publication Data

The nature of cities / edited by Andrew C. Isenberg.
p. cm. — (Studies in comparative history, ISSN 1539-4905 ; v. 8)
Includes bibliographical references and index.
ISBN 1-58046-220-0 (hardcover : alk. paper)
1. Cities and towns—United States—History. 2. Venice (Italy)—History. 3. London (England)—History. 4. Urban ecology—History. 5. Urban health—History. I. Isenberg, Andrew C. (Andrew Christian) II. Series.
HT123.n35 2005
307.76'0973—dc22

2005018083

A catalogue record for this title is available from the British Library.

This publication is printed on acid-free paper.

Cover image: Eleanor McClatchy Collection, City of Sacramento, History and Science Division, Sacramento Archives and Museum Collection Center.

Cover design by Adam B. Bohannon

For
Arthur F. McEvoy

Contents

Acknowledgments

This book emerged from a conference in December 2003, at the Shelby Cullom Davis Center for Historical Studies at Princeton University. The authors in this volume are grateful to the Davis Center for its sponsorship of the conference and of this collection. We thank especially the Davis Center's director, Gyan Prakash, and its manager, Jennifer Houle. We also wish to thank Sarah Elkind, David Freund, Kevin Kruse, Neil Maher, and Peter Siskind for their constructive criticism.

Introduction

New Directions in Urban Environmental History

Andrew C. Isenberg

When environmental history emerged as a new field twenty-five years ago, its practitioners were concerned primarily with the history of rural and wild places. This emphasis on the countryside reflected environmental history's genealogy in the study of frontiers, agricultural history, and the idea of nature. The study of the North American frontier had a significant influence on the development of environmental history. The late nineteenth- and early twentieth-century historian Frederick Jackson Turner's study of the transformation of the western "wilderness" has been particularly important; the historian William Cronon has characterized much of environmental history, defined as "the story of human beings working with changing tools to transform the resources of the land," as fundamentally "Turnerian in its implications."[1] Part of that Turnerian inheritance has been the notion of opposition between city and countryside; in Turner's frontier paradigm, as one grows, the other must recede.

Yet environmental history has never been so facile as to be simply derived from Turner. The field has drawn much of its methodological inspiration and theoretical sophistication from the *Annales* historians of mid-twentieth-century France. The *Annalistes* conceived of a "total history" that eschewed the ephemera of politics and culture in favor of analyzing the deeper, material roots of social structure in climate, geography, and the production of agricultural commodities. As the historian Donald Worster has argued, the *Annales* approach found one of its fullest and most profound expressions in environmental history, which is perhaps the epitome of grassroots history.[2] In 1990, Worster drew on the *Annales* agrarian historiography to propose that environmental history's research agenda should be "agroecological."[3]

Environmental history's inheritance derives as much from intellectual and cultural history as from material history. Yet here too circumstances directed environmental historians toward a focus on rural and wild places. In the late 1940s and early 1950s, first in the United States (particularly in American studies departments) and then elsewhere, cultural and intellectual historians produced a number of studies of wilderness and nature. The first generation of American studies scholars saw in the wilderness the roots of American cultural identity. Writing in the early 1980s, the environmental historian Richard White declared that "wilderness has become the highway to the American psyche most favored by intellectual historians."[4] In short, whether they drew their inspiration from cultural history or from material history, the first generation of environmental historians focused primarily on wilderness and agriculture.

In the first decade and a half after the field emerged, only a few environmental historians concentrated on urban places. These historians have consistently criticized the broader field's focus on farms and wilderness. Worster has been a favorite target for critics, from his advocacy of "agroecology" to his explicit rejection of cities as part of environmental history: "The built environment is wholly expressive of culture; its study is already well advanced in the history of architecture, technology, and the city," he wrote in 1988. "When we step beyond the self-reflecting world of humankind to encounter the nonhuman sphere, environmental history finds its main themes of study."[5]

Yet in one sense the criticism of Worster is misplaced; he did not invent the intellectual divide between city and countryside. Rather, at a time when few historians bothered to consider the agency and presence of the nonhuman natural world, he took on the study of a largely neglected subject. Indeed, the disinterest of Worster and other environmental historians in urban places was equally matched by urban historians' long-standing disregard for the natural environment. Lewis Mumford, one of the early leaders of the field of urban studies, captured this perspective when he wrote in 1938, "as the pavement spreads, nature is pushed away."[6] Except for the study of epidemics and urban parks, urban historians working in the decades following Mumford's pronouncement did little to contradict him.[7]

Yet beneath the formal divide between environmental and urban history, considerable informal intellectual borrowing persisted. Each field adopted theoretical constructs from the other. Although most early scholars of urban studies ignored nonhuman nature within and without the bounds of the city, they borrowed liberally from the environmental sciences to conceptualize cities. In the first decades of the twentieth century, the Chicago School of urban sociologists articulated the idea of the city as an evolving organism and borrowed the concept of human ecology to track the growth of urban space and the activities of city residents. Robert E. Park, a University of Chicago sociologist, wrote in 1915 that while the urban "geometrical form suggests that the city is a purely artificial construction," in fact the city only "seems" to be "mere artifact." Park argued that "as a whole, the city is a growth."[8] Park, other Chicago School sociologists, and their notion of the city as an organism dominated urban studies in the early twentieth century.

The earliest urban environmental historians—such estimable scholars as Martin Melosi and Joel Tarr—took their historiographical cues from the Chicago School. Their work's focus on problems of industrial pollution and urban sanitation revealed the influence of the model of the urban organism. Melosi, for instance, while rejecting the most extreme versions of organism theory, has opted for a more technologically refined version of it: "the idea of the city as a system." Similarly, Tarr, while insisting on the distinction between cities and the nonhuman natural environment, has adopted some of the terminology of the Chicago School; he titled a recent article on sanitation, resource consumption, and pollution in Pittsburgh "The Metabolism of the Industrial City." In the essay, Tarr invoked the ecologist Eugene Odum's characterization of the city as a "parasite."[9] These historians' arm's-length embrace of Chicago School ideas demonstrates the potential and well as the pitfalls of the organism model: it is a useful tool for thought, yet when applied to specific places and times, like all theoretical models its tidy precision breaks down.

A more pernicious problem inherent in the undiluted form of the organism model is its tendency to obscure the power relations that are central to urban history. The scholar who has dealt most ably with this problem is Andrew Hurley, whose masterful study of Gary, Indiana, synthesized the city-as-organism school's interest in urban pollution with urban history's long-standing concern with residential discrimination. Gary's growth as a steel town polluted the air, water, and soil, yet beginning in the late 1940s, middle-class whites distanced themselves from the worst industrial pollution by removing to Gary's suburbs. African Americans, meanwhile, had few options but to remain in neighborhoods nearest the plants.[10]

Unlike Melosi, Tarr, and Hurley, most environmental historians have studied the rural rather than the urban, yet much of their scholarship nonetheless has had a decidedly metropolitan perspective: urbanites consumed both peripheral natural resources as commodities and wilderness as a recreational amenity. Historians such as William Cronon, in his study of nineteenth-century Chicago's consumption of timber, cattle, and grain, have demonstrated how as a source of commodities or as idealized nature, the environment felt the imprint of urban society.[11]

Even in Cronon's widely read work, the influence of the urban organism model remains. Cronon drew much of his theoretical inspiration from central place theory, a body of thought that originated with the early nineteenth-century geographer Johann Heinrich von Thünen.[12] Central place theory imagines the city at the center of concentric rings of dependent rural economic activities; with profitable, perishable goods (for instance, orchards and dairy production) in the ring closest to the center; and the production of cheap products in bulk (such as wheat cultivation) in the outermost ring.

This formulation, which Cronon has described as "more rhetorical than analytical" in his thinking, has its virtues as a way to conceptualize the human organization of space; not least of all, in using it Cronon managed to synthesize urban and agricultural history. Nonetheless, central place theory is effectively the organism model of urban geographers writ large. Like the organism model, central place theory tends not only toward an idealization of the city but toward a masking of power relations. Cronon's Chicago absorbed resources from the hinterlands and transformed them into commodities. His study pays relatively little attention to the stockyard and lumbermill workers who effected those transformations, yet benefited little from doing so.

Cronon has defended his exclusion of class, social, and labor history from his analysis, writing that *Nature's Metropolis* "was already threatening to sprawl in too many directions." That defense echoed Worster's onetime call for excluding the study of cities from environmental history. Worster had feared that the research agenda of urbanists would overwhelm the study of nonhuman nature. Likewise, Cronon chose to exclude class and labor history from *Nature's Metropolis* rather than see them, as he once put it, "trump all other analytical categories"—including nature.[13] His silence on these subjects demonstrates environmental historians' wariness of synthesis with class history a decade and a half ago—an indication of a subfield still then emerging and afraid of being overwhelmed by more established fields.

The essays in this volume benefit from building on the work of Cronon and Worster as well as Tarr, Melosi, and others. No longer concerned with proving the relevance of urban places to environmental history, no longer beholden to the organism or central place models of urban studies, no longer afraid that environmental history will be subsumed by other fields through greater attention to social, labor, or cultural history, the essays in this collection mark a new direction in urban environmental history. The contributions to this volume draw on scholarly literature on race, class, consumerism, landscape studies, and the body to deal with such questions as racial and class conflicts in urban public spaces; the cultural construction and control of public spaces by economic and government powers; and the idealization of cities as separate from nature. The methodology of the contributors is syncretic, combining an interest in cultural history with urban and environmental historians' long-standing focus on the material world.

The volume began as a conference, "The Nature of Cities: New Perspectives in Urban Environmental History," at the Shelby Cullom Davis Center for Historical Studies at Princeton University, 12–13 December 2003. The contributors explored the intersection of cities and the natural environment from a variety of analytical perspectives, in an array of places, including New York, San Francisco, London, New Orleans, Venice, and Seattle, across a broad period from the seventeenth century to the present. The book is divided into three parts. The four essays in the first part, "Urban Spaces, Death, and the Body," are social and cultural histories of epidemics, urban pollution, and death in major commercial and industrial cities in the nineteenth and twentieth centuries. Race figures prominently in these chapters. In New Orleans in 1853, a yellow fever epidemic claimed ten thousand lives; 90 percent of the victims were white. According to Ari Kelman, surviving whites conflated their fears of the epidemic with their fears of an urban slave rebellion. In San Francisco in the first decade of the twentieth century, as Joanna Dyl explains, city officials initially racialized bubonic plague as a disease of Chinese immigrants. Ellen Stroud analyzes how in Harlem in the late twentieth century, African Americans protested against the presence in their community of a crematorium that processed the bodies of wealthy Manhattanites. Class differences also figure in each of these conflicts, as well as in late nineteenth-century London, where, according to Peter Thorsheim, parks for working-class citizens, developed on former prison grounds, like those jails served as a means of social control. Together, the chapters in the first part share a number of concerns, foremost among which are how death and dying inverted racial and class hierarchies and upset notions of what was considered natural. Key to each of these essays is the emerging literature on the body. These chapters explore how fears of disease and degeneration in the city fixated on the bodies of urban inhabitants.

While the chapters in the first part largely focus inward on city inhabitants, the chapters in the second part, "The Geography of Power and Consumption," take into account cities' relationships to the land and water surrounding and penetrating them. As Karl Appuhn explains, in seventeenth-century Venice, advocates of flood control and reclamation schemes squared off against each other; at issue was whether Venice would be a commercial city facing the sea or the capital of an inland agricultural empire. In nineteenth-century Sacramento, California, city officials also engaged in extensive flood control projects. As in Venice, officials in Sacramento looked not only to the economic prospects of the city but also to their own political futures. They were concerned with both protecting their investments in city property and, by building politically popular levees, establishing their political legitimacy. While these two essays focus on municipal politics, in twentieth-century Seattle, according to Matthew Klingle, merchants and boosters drew on the emerging consumer economy to promote the city as a capital of outdoor recreation. Challenging the static and deterministic central place and city-as-organism models of urban historians, these chapters show the economic and political calculations that constructed cities and the regions surrounding them. In Venice, Sacramento, and Seattle, cities reshaped their hinterlands but the urban periphery was not merely passive. Hinterlands shaped cities as well: natural catastrophes heightened tensions between opposing forces in the cities.

The chapters in the third part, "Cities Deconstructed," focus on the cultural and ecological tenuousness of urban places. In southern Africa, as Emmanuel Kreike demonstrates, the populations of Ovamboland dispersed under the pressure of European colonization. Eventually, such depopulated places were incorporated into national parks. In postwar France, regional development planners reversed the centuries-long trend toward the concentration of economic and political power in Paris. To decentralize a central place required that regional metropolitan centers have hinterlands of their own; to create just such a regional hinterland for Lyon, French planners pressed the Rhône River into service, damming it and diverting it for power and irrigation. In short, the chapters in this final section historicize the rise and fall of cities.

One common denominator of the chapters in this volume is a concern with power: political power, imperial power, and the power of historians, archaeologists, geographers, and others to shape our understanding of past and present landscapes. In Sacramento in the 1850s, it was the power of the city government over squatters. In Seattle, it was the city's power to force poor fishers and squatters from urban parks. In San Francisco in 1907, it was the power of a municipal government to concretize the city, and to expel chicken farmers and dairy producers. As Joanna Dyl makes clear, the burden of sanitizing the city fell most heavily on those least able to afford it: the working poor who kept chickens or eked out an existence selling manure from city stables to farmers in the countryside. Modernization was thus neither a neutral nor an apolitical process, but one that reflected the maldistribution of wealth and power in the city.

In postwar France, the Fourth Republic, reflecting the provincial Vichy regime's resentments against Paris, pushed through a regional development plan that shifted economic resources to the periphery. Sara Pritchard shows how advocates of regional development drew on long-standing provincial antiurban feeling to characterize the dominance of Paris in France as akin to a disease in the French body. Likewise, Emmanuel Kreike highlights the power of archaeologists and geographers to minimize the significance of former urban settlements in places that Europeans colonized. European conquest forced the abandonment of cities and villages in Africa; colonists culturally constructed abandoned places as wilderness. He suggests that the caricature of precolonial Africa as a wild or rural landscape devoid of dense settlements was and continues to be an effort to legitimize European colonization.

Another common concern of the authors is to *historicize* the development and the decline of cities. Joanna Dyl shows how San Francisco's relationship with its hinterland in the aftermath of the earthquake was complex: to combat plague, the municipal government exiled the poultry and dairy industries to the countryside. Her work suggests that the neat concentric model of central place theoreticians is not an inevitable natural condition (a sort of "climax theory" for the urban organism) but rather the result of catastrophe and the exercise of political power. Sara Pritchard's chapter shows a different kind of exercise of political power: the reapportionment of economic and political capital away from Paris, France's center of gravity, and toward smaller cities orbiting on the periphery. Her study of the Rhône region is the counterpart of Karl Appuhn's chapter on sixteenth- and seventeenth-century Venice. Venetian leaders had declined to develop the interior in favor of a seaward orientation of their commercial empire. In twentieth-century Marseille, decolonization forced French planners to turn their gaze from the Mediterranean to the interior.

At the same time that the contributors to this volume historicize cities, they challenge linear narratives in urban and environmental history. Emmanuel Kreike directly challenges the idea of a European-led progression from rural wilderness to civilization. He both blurs the distinction between the categories of rural and urban and argues that cities not only rise but also fall. Conversely, Sacramento and San Francisco averted collapse after flood, earthquake, and plague by imposing citification—an implicit admission that such development had failed to progress on its own. In postwar France, peripheral cities rose up against the metropolitan center and demanded a greater share of economic and political power. In all of these cases the cultural constructedness and physical tenuousness of cities looms large. Here is where urban and environmental histories intersect: both fields teach us that nature and cities alike are constructed and changeable.

These changes and constructions derived from unequally held power, and resulted in unequally divided benefits. New Orleans's slaves, London and San Francisco's working poor, Harlem's African Americans, squatters in Seattle and Sacramento, and the dispossessed San of southern Africa bore an unequal share of the costs of urban and environmental change. So too did the waters of Venice, the Rhône and Sacramento rivers, and the air over New York City, among other places. Yet the environment was an actor as well as acted upon: flood, earthquake, and disease testified to the agency and presence of nature in urban history.

NOTES

1. Frederick Jackson Turner, "The Significance of the Frontier in American History," American Historical Association *Annual Report* (1893): 199–227; William Cronon, "Revisiting the Vanishing Frontier: The Legacy of Fredrick Jackson Turner," *Western Historical Quarterly* 18 (April 1987): 157–76.

2. For an analysis of the influence of the *Annales* school on the development of environmental history, see Andrew C. Isenberg, "Historicizing Natural Environments: The Deep Roots of Environmental History," in *A Companion to Western Historical Thought,* ed. Lloyd Kramer and Sarah Maza (Oxford: Blackwell, 2002), pp. 372–89; see also Donald Worster, "Doing Environmental History," in *The Ends of the Earth: Perspectives on Modern Environmental History,* ed. Worster (New York: Cambridge University Press, 1988), pp. 289–307.

3. Worster, "Transformations of the Earth: Toward an Agroecological Perspective in History," *Journal of American History* 76 (March 1990): 1087–1106.

4. Richard White, "American Environmental History: The Development of a New Historical Field," *Pacific Historical Review* 54 (1985): 297–335. White referred to Roderick Nash, *Wilderness and the American Mind* (New Haven, Conn.: Yale University Press, 1967); Leo Marx, *The Machine in the Garden: Technology and the Pastoral Ideal in America* (New York: Oxford University Press, 1964); and Henry Nash Smith, *Virgin Land: The American West as Symbol and Myth* (Cambridge, Mass.: Harvard University Press, 1950), among others. In European historiography, the exemplar of cultural studies of nature is Keith Thomas, *Man and the Natural World: A History of Modern Sensibility* (New York: Pantheon, 1983).

5. Worster, "Doing Environmental History," p. 293. For criticism of Worster, see Jonathan J. Keyes, "A Place of Its Own: Urban Environmental History," *Journal of Urban History* 26 (March 2000): 380–90; Joel Tarr and Christine Rosen, 'The Environment and the City," ibid., 20 (May 1994): 299–310.

6. Lewis Mumford, *The Culture of Cities* (1938; San Diego: Harcourt Brace, 1970), p. 253, quoted in Ari Kelman, *A River and Its City: The Nature of Landscape in New Orleans* (Berkeley: University of California Press, 2003), p. 8.

7. The classic study of disease in the city is Charles Rosenberg, *The Cholera Years: The United States in 1832, 1849, and 1866* (Chicago: University of Chicago Press, 1962). See also Richard J. Evans, *Death In Hamburg: Society and Politics in the Cholera Years* (Oxford: Oxford University Press, 1987). For urban parks, see David Schuyler, *The New Urban Landscape: The Redefinition of City Form in Nineteenth-Century America* (Baltimore: Johns Hopkins University Press, 1986).

8. Robert E. Park, "The City: Suggestions for the Investigation of Human Behavior in the City Environment," *American Journal of Sociology* 20 (March 1915): 577–612. For the city as an organism, see also Louis Wirth, "Human Ecology," *American Journal of Sociology* 50 (July 1945): 483–88; Amos Hawley, *Human Ecology: A Theory of Community Structure* (New York: Ronald Press, 1950); Spenser Havlick, *The Urban Organism: The City's Natural Resources from an Environmental Perspective* (New York: Macmillan, 1974); Graeme Davison, "The City as Natural System: Theories of Urban Society in Early Nineteenth-Century Britain," in *The Pursuit of Urban History,* ed. Derek Fraser and Anthony Sutcliffe (London, 1983).

9. See Martin Melosi, *The Sanitary City: Urban Infrastructure in America from Colonial Times to the Present* (Baltimore: Johns Hopkins University Press, 2000), pp. 2–8. See also Melosi's "The Place of the City in Environmental History," *Environmental History Review* 17 (Spring 1993): 1–24. See also Joel Tarr, "The Metabolism of the Industrial City: The Case of Pittsburgh," *Journal of Urban History* 28 (July 2002): 511–545; and Tarr, *The Search for the Ultimate Sink: Urban Pollution in Historical Perspective* (Akron, Ohio: University of Akron Press, 1996). See also Eugene Odum, *Ecology and Our Endangered Life Support Systems* (Sunderland, Mass.: Sinauer Associates, 1989), p. 17.

10. Andrew Hurley, *Environmental Inequalities: Race, Class, and Industrial Pollution in Gary, Indiana, 1945–1980* (Chapel Hill: University of North Carolina Press, 1995).

11. William Cronon, *Nature's Metropolis: Chicago and the Great West* (New York: Norton, 1991). See also Peter J. Schmitt, *Back to Nature: The Arcadian Myth in Urban America* (New York: Oxford University Press, 1969).

12. Johann Heinrich von Thünen, *Von Thünen's Isolated State,* ed. Peter Hall (1826; New York: Pergamon Press, 1966).

13. See Mary Beth Pudup et al., "William Cronon's *Nature's Metropolis:* A Symposium," *Antipode* 26 (April 1994): 113–76. Cronon's reply deals capably and persuasively with the *Antipode* critiques—a job made easier by some of his critics' over-the-top polemicism.

Part I

Urban Spaces, Death, and the Body

I

New Orleans's Phantom Slave Insurrection of 1853

Racial Anxiety, Urban Ecology, and Human Bodies as Public Spaces

Ari Kelman

The Rebellion

As the cathedral bell on Jackson Square rang out 11 P.M. on 13 June 1853, George Wright, a disheveled *homme libre de couleur* (free man of color) stumbled through the door of New Orleans's police station and demanded to see someone about a matter of great consequence. Wright then related an elaborate plan for a slave insurrection that would begin just hours later, sometime before dawn. The incredulous lieutenant who received the report barely paid attention to the details. Still, because a slave rebellion, no matter how improbable, was serious business, the lieutenant reluctantly summoned the chief of police, Stephen O'Leary. The skeptical chief later recalled that he, too, had listened impatiently at first. Only after Wright offered to bring the police to one of the insurrection's ringleaders did O'Leary seriously consider that the alarming tale could possibly be true, or at least worth investigating.[1]

Wright then led the way through New Orleans's streets to the rebellion's headquarters. Police officers later recounted that the man Wright met was "loaded with weapons—a moving arsenal. He had a knife, a cavalry saber, a six-barreled revolver, loaded and capped, a bag of bullets, about a pound of powder, and two boxes of percussion caps." As he was interrogated, the jailed conspirator related a startling story. There were at least twenty-five hundred men, made up of free people of color, slaves, and sympathetic whites, stationed throughout New Orleans. This army of liberation stood ready to occupy the city's arsenals, the heavily fortified U.S. Mint, and other public buildings, all of which would be used as beachheads in the ensuing battles for control of New Orleans. Agents of the conspiracy waiting throughout the city would then torch the town, signaling to an invading force of slaves, thousands strong, poised to descend in a fury upon New Orleans from surrounding plantations. With the gateway to the Mississippi firmly in its grasp, the rebellion would spread upriver throughout the South, inevitably putting an end to slavery once and for all. (Students of the antebellum era will notice striking parallels with John Brown's raid on Harper's Ferry, at the time still more than five years in the future.)[2]

Although Chief O'Leary remained uncertain about the conspiracy's existence, he nonetheless contacted Mayor A. D. Crossman, who, in turn, spread the alarm to the commander of the Southwestern District of the U.S. Army, Major General D. E. Twiggs. With the promise of armed reinforcements ready to come to the city's aid if need be, Crossman and O'Leary then deployed the entire police force to patrol New Orleans's deserted streets, ordered that all people of color seen outdoors be apprehended immediately, and sent word to neighboring plantation owners to be on the lookout for "suspicious characters and for anything unusual among the slaves." With so many safeguards in place, the mayor and police chief hunkered down for the night, which passed without any further incidents.[3]

By the next morning, it had become clear to many New Orleanians that what was widely being called the "Negro effervescence" had been little more than a hoax, as one journalist raged, a product of the "twisted mind of a deluded" free person of color. Summing up what seemed to be the prevailing mood in the city that day, a merchant wrote in his ledger book that "the matter passed by with little notice as being too foolish or ridiculous for belief—and in a few hours was only mentioned jestingly." The local press, eager to reassure skittish New Orleanians, as well as wary traders and investors throughout the region, did what it could to spread the word that all was well. One article employed rhetoric that was fast becoming familiar as the nation's sectional crisis deepened: "depraved whites who deliberately speculate for dishonest gain upon the ignorance, credibility and excitability of the Negro" incited "insurrections and insubordinations," the *Daily Picayune* suggested. Although today such stories read like collective whistling in the dark, the message then was heartfelt and clear: slaves were happy with their lot; it was outsiders, most likely abolitionists, who poisoned race relations in the South.[4]

Still, despite the press's efforts and the fact that the insurrection never amounted to more than rumors, widespread fears in the city could not be allayed so easily, as talk of the rebellion persisted for months afterward. It seems that New Orleanians remained uneasy that their chattel and the city's free people of color, with help from troublemaking whites, might rise up together against the local slaveocracy. Numbers provide some context for this stubborn paranoia. There were approximately ten thousand *gens* (people) *de couleur libres* living in New Orleans in 1853, accounting for just under 10 percent of the city's population, and a slightly greater number of slaves. Statistics, though, do not entirely account for the lingering worries about the rebellion. Nor do census figures explain why concerned citizens and city officials continued to demand that free and enslaved people of color not be allowed to walk the streets after dark, that businesses ("Negro groggeries") serving alcohol to *gens de couleur libres* be shuttered immediately, and that all slaves with reputations for violence or even insolence be locked up.[5]

To get to the root of the rumors about the rebellion one must look closely at New Orleans's environmental history. Because the insurrection took place (or, more accurately, did not take place) as a massive yellow fever epidemic hit the city and ultimately killed approximately ten thousand people in just six months, local whites were more sensitive than usual to rumors of racial unrest in New Orleans. As the outbreak—which a leading historian of public health has called the "worst single epidemic ever to strike an American city"[6]—prostrated New Orleans's power structure, white elites feared that members of the city's huge enslaved and free African-American communities could lash out at their oppressors with relative impunity. The pervasive concerns about a slave rebellion in the city thus seem predictable, even justifiable, in retrospect. This essay will argue that the coincidence of the epidemic and phantom insurrection in New Orleans underscores the social implications of urban ecology for the dynamics, depth, and impact of racial anxiety.

More significant than the rumored insurrection itself was the manner in which the city's racial anxiety manifested itself during the summer of 1853. As New Orleanians grappled with the ravages of the epidemic, and struggled to cope with their ongoing concerns about race relations in the city, time and again they focused on corporeal issues, on how bodies were reacting to conditions around them. Whites in the city, especially, became fascinated with the perceived workings of embodied racial and ethnic difference. When disease and panic began transforming social hierarchies in the city, New Orleanians focused on what they thought of as the very nature of blackness and whiteness: phenotypic responses to environmental stimuli, literally the way that bodies changed in the face of illness. Many of these discussions focused on people at work and at rest, as laboring bodies and the thousands of corpses that were yellow fever's most gruesome by-product became focal points for the city's concerns during the summer of 1853. Ultimately, the outbreak and the racial anxiety it prompted altered the urban fabric in New Orleans, emptying some usually crowded landscapes of people, filling others with bodies seemingly out of place, and in the process tampering with the local population's perceptions of the divide between public and private spaces.

The Epidemic

Three weeks before George Wright walked through the door of New Orleans's police station to announce that the city's people of color would rise up and lead a crusade to crush slavery throughout the South, the first victim of the great yellow fever epidemic of 1853 succumbed to the disease. Within just a few days of that small tragedy, which passed virtually unnoticed at the time, several more people, all of whom had recently arrived in the city, died of the same cause. By the end of May, alert doctors at New Orleans's Charity Hospital were increasingly alarmed by the sudden influx of patients all sharing similar symptoms: sustained high fevers, debilitating head and body aches, painful sensitivity to light, and, in several instances, jaundice. As a result of this constellation of cases, a group of physicians conferred and decided to perform an autopsy on one of the recently deceased men. What they found in the victim's stomach, "two ounces of the black vomit," confirmed their worst fears. In an era in which yellow fever could be difficult to distinguish from a host of other inscrutable illnesses, the presence of vomit stained by blood was as close to a definitive diagnostic tool as doctors had at their disposal. It seemed that yellow fever was loose in the city.[7]

In the weeks after the fateful autopsy, even as the press denied that an epidemic had gripped New Orleans, several hundred more people died of yellow fever. The disease's presence thus provided a grim backdrop when Chief O'Leary and Mayor Crossman heard news of the proposed slave rebellion. Both men, despite the litany of daily press denials, knew of the epidemic's seriousness because of reports they were receiving from Charity Hospital, and both knew how precarious the situation had become. If New Orleans's people of color rose up with yellow fever already running rampant, the city might never recover. Even if the rebellion failed, news of racial violence, particularly when coupled with rumors of pestilence, would cause a mass exodus from the city, as residents and traders lit out for safer locales. The coincidence of two such dire threats to the social and economic order likely contributed to the gravity with which Crossman and O'Leary treated Wright's story. Still, a question lingers: Why did New Orleanians remain concerned about the insurrection for so long despite the local press's and municipal government's efforts? The answer, again, can be traced to the disease attacking the city, especially because of the odd way yellow fever seemed to behave during the epidemic of 1853. The virus attacked sections of New Orleans previously deemed safe and bodies long thought immune.[8]

Over the previous four decades, major yellow fever epidemics—ones in which more than one hundred people died—had struck New Orleans at least every third year, so the city was used to coping with illness on a grand scale. Consequently, many New Orleanians had accommodated themselves to periodic outbreaks, not just because of past experiences, but also due to a host of medical misconceptions that swirled around yellow fever, urban spaces, and white bodies. Mid-nineteenth-century physicians knew little about yellow fever's origins or mode of transmission, believing that the disease, like other scourges, was spawned by conditions specific to particular locales and transmitted by miasmas, vapors rising from swamps or rotting organic matter.

The city's doctors then built dangerous conclusions atop this shaky foundation, suggesting that yellow fever could not spread from one place to another. The disease, in sum, was neither portable nor contagious. So, while New Orleans, surrounded by swamps, dotted with markets where produce decomposed in the sun, and plagued by bad drainage and heavy rain, had to guard against miasmas, yellow fever could at least be expected to have a predictable geography. The disease would strike filthy parts of the city, leaving cleaner spots unscathed.[9] Other myths, about the interaction of white bodies and the environment, also had consoled longtime residents of New Orleans during past outbreaks and seemed to offer some solace early in the epidemic of 1853. In July, for instance, as the press belatedly admitted that yellow fever had arrived in the city, the *Delta* reported, "attacks of the malady are confined exclusively to strangers." This assertion emerged out of a half-baked notion, drawn from a recipe of equal parts flawed empiricism and cultural conceit, which suggested that Creoles (this protean term will be used here as it was most commonly in mid-nineteenth-century New Orleans, to mean Louisiana-born white citizens) and so-called acclimated people were immune to yellow fever because of prolonged exposure to the local environs. In other words, in 1853, many New Orleanians believed that ties to the Delta's unusual environment fostered immunity to disease by bringing bodies into concert with the city's otherwise hazardous surroundings.[10]

There may have been at least some truth lurking behind these otherwise misguided claims. In most yellow fever epidemics, well over half of the people who contracted the disease lived, and, as with other viruses (measles or chicken pox, for example) those who survived were immune for the rest of their lives. The probable explanation for apparent group immunity, thus, was actually that many New Orleanians had weathered a mild bout with the virus—often during childhood in the case of Creoles—though few knew it, as misdiagnoses were common. Blessed with a survivor's immunity, they never sickened as adults, and often lived out their lives certain that cultural superiority and deep roots in the city shielded them from illness.[11]

Popular belief in Creole immunity and acclimation not only comforted many white New Orleanians during outbreaks but also became pillars of eth nic and class identity. Because health in the face of sickness ostensibly was a product of a body's ties to the environment, immune New Orleanians believed their heartiness provided membership in a privileged social category. Such ideas emerged from and strengthened currents of class conflict and xenophobia in the city. Immune New Orleanians blamed victims of outbreaks for their plight, arguing that the dead and dying had brought sickness on themselves through bad habits or disrespect for the environment. In 1853, for instance, the press noted of immigrants and the working classes: they "congregate in damp and unwholesome places, and what with exposure, neglect and want, become the first victims of an epidemic." Years later, satirist and social critic George Washington Cable poked fun at Creoles for these attitudes about yellow fever. Cable explained that the Creole "had, and largely retains still, an absurd belief in his entire immunity from attack. When he has it, it is something else. As for strangers—he threw up his palms and eyebrows—nobody asked them to come to New Orleans." At the time, though, in an era marked by nativism nationwide, epidemics offered environmental justifications for anti-immigrant and class prejudice, and provided immune New Orleanians with a misplaced notion of cultural superiority and false security.[12]

The problem with these theories became clear at the end of July 1853, as more than a thousand people died from yellow fever in the month's last two weeks. The shocking mortality rate left white observers of all classes and ethnicities terrified and increasingly anxious about their bodies, as the virus shattered time-tested myths in the city. New Orleanians had long counted on what appeared to be yellow fever's consistent behavior: the disease thrived only in filthy areas, amidst newcomers and the working classes. In 1853, though, yellow fever struck throughout town and cut across the social strata, leading one doctor to note that after "gaining strength by what it fed upon, it began to travel to other and more distant points, to extend its arms, so to speak, in every direction." Then, the disease seemingly developed new potency, causing an observer to warn that it had "acquired strength to attack those who consider themselves impregnable." In short, even bodies of Creoles and longtime New Orleanians proved vulnerable to yellow fever in 1853, which challenged the assumptions of some members of these groups about ethnicity and class prerogatives. So oddly did the virus act that a trader wrote: "the nature of the disease is universally admitted to be different from former types." As fear spread, rumors circulated that the city faced not yellow fever, but the Black Death.[13]

With hindsight and some knowledge of epidemiology as a guide, it is clear that the virus actually behaved normally in 1853, capitalizing on New Orleans's urban ecology. For example, despite claims to the contrary, yellow fever was contagious; it was transmitted by female *Aedes aegypti* mosquitoes. When one of these insects took a blood meal—as often as twelve times in a month—from an infected host, she gathered nourishment for her eggs as well as a dose of the virus. Once a carrier, she transmitted the disease each time she fed throughout her life, like a flying dirty needle, randomly infecting unsuspecting victims for as long as two months. Originally from Africa, *Aedes aegypti* came to the Americas as a by-product of the international slave trade, often labeled a kind of "biological revenge" by scholars eager to find morality in the workings of the nonhuman world. New Orleans provided an especially welcoming home for these bugs, because of features of its built environment and climate. Warm temperatures and high humidity suited *Aedes aegypti,* and, over time, the mosquitoes adapted to city life, where crowds of people provided self-serve buffets. Female *Aedes aegypti* also preferred laying eggs in artificial containers, and through the first half of the nineteenth century, most New Orleanians took drinking water from cisterns "in close proximity" to their homes.[14]

Because of these conditions, linked both to the city's natural and to its built environments, 1853 proved to be a banner year for mosquitoes. In early June, with yellow fever already loose in the streets, writhing clouds of mosquitoes literally darkened the dusk skies above New Orleans. L. H. Webb, a student who found "the mosquitoes troublesome," confessed to his diary that he spent a week fruitlessly trying to drive them from his home with cigar smoke. After fouling his nest, he gave up and "went to bed considerably nauseated." Webb's troubles were relatively common throughout New Orleans, and by the end of the month, journalists were chronicling the infestation in articles printed next to gossip about the conspiracy brewing among the city's people of color. A writer at the *Daily Delta,* for example, noted, "we have never known the mosquitoes to be half as severe as they are at present." In a tragic example of historical irony, however, he celebrated the infestation, insisting that pestilence would not visit New Orleans during the coming summer "for the simple reason that Providence does not afflict us with two curses at one and the same time; and, to add yellow fever to the present terrible visitation of mosquitoes, would be too much for human endurance."[15]

So in 1853 yellow fever terrified New Orleanians, partly because they did not know that the disease was contagious or that it was carried by an insect vector. Still more threatening, though, illness was ignoring ostensibly fixed social and spatial boundaries in the city. As yellow fever traveled on *Aedes aegypti's* wings, it transgressed borders dividing one section of New Orleans from the next. It spread citywide without regard to labels people fixed to urban landscapes: filthy or pure, elite or common, even public or private. Such categories proved meaningless to organisms moving through space constructed not socially, but ecologically. A mosquito might bite an immigrant living in a flophouse near the river, fly a short distance inland to the ornate home of a wealthy Creole merchant, and pass along the virus while taking its next blood meal. When yellow fever traveled through the city in this way, it rendered even the most private spaces public, and, by moving from one person to the next, regardless of a victim's social standing or ethnicity, did the same to bodies of the people who contracted the disease. As a result, New Orleanians who had always counted themselves immune based on prosperity, breeding, ties to the Delta, or clean living, were shocked when they sickened.

Perhaps more even than the fast-rising death count, this reworking of private spaces, including elite bodily spaces, prompted panic in late July of 1853. Private places are desirable in cities, in part because they are perceived to be refuges from the bustle and apparent danger of urban living. These spaces are considered relatively safe and subject to individual control rather than group negotiation. By this definition, bodies are the quintessential private spaces in metropolitan settings. During periods of stress in cities, such as epidemics or rumors of street violence, private spaces become more valuable, particularly if disease or danger supposedly only strikes disorderly or impure landscapes. In such instances control of one's spatial environment can literally mean the difference between life and death. As a result, early in the summer of 1853, wealthy New Orleanians, along with Creoles and the acclimated, relied on the perceived safety of their homes and the impregnability of their bodies, which were supposed to be isolated from the filthiest parts of the city, ostensibly beyond the reach of yellow fever and therefore safe. When circumstances proved otherwise, when yellow fever stripped away some of the features associated with private space, panic ensued.

By late July, spreading fear about the consequences of the outbreak provided the context in which many New Orleanians still fretted about the loyalty of the city's people of color. New Orleans was facing its worst epidemic on record, as yellow fever broke rules it had made over the years; close to fifteen hundred citizens had died and thousands of others had fled the city, leaving streets deserted and markets abandoned; and even Creoles and longstanding New Orleanians worried about their health, as elite white bodies, stricken by a disease usually associated with common people and immigrants, broke down. The city's social, economic, and spatial orders were under attack, as yellow fever killed more people in more districts every day, exacerbating racial anxiety, a part of daily life in New Orleans under the best of circumstances. Adding to the city's fear and sense of vulnerability, and likely one of the major reasons New Orleanians were so concerned about the local communities of color, most doctors believed African Americans were immune to yellow fever, and nothing during the epidemic of 1853 suggested otherwise. In sum, as New Orleans's power structure lay in a shambles, devastated by illness, the city's people of color were healthy and perhaps still hatching plans for a rebellion.[16]

YELLOW FEVER, BLACK BODIES

In August 1853, yellow fever inscribed itself deeply onto New Orleans's landscapes and population, further altering the municipal social order and increasing the already high level of racial anxiety in the city. At the time, thousands of sickly citizens bore the disease's signature on their haunted faces: a yellowish tint that caused even friends to back away in horror. As yellow fever reconstituted white bodies in this way, it shifted New Orleanians' senses of themselves and the ways other perceived them. Even mild illness can alter people's perceptions of their bodies. Fever can cause shaking, a cough can make one consider each breath taken into the lungs, and violent sneezing can punctuate a day. In each case, involuntary muscle movements, which are usually ignored, become manifest and troubling. The sense of corporeal change and related vulnerability in late summer 1853 was far more extreme, as yellow fever literally made white bodies colorful. And in a city like New Orleans, whose complicated racial categories had more in common with parts of Latin America—where subtle shades of color mattered far more than in the typically biracial United States—jaundice thus not only trumpeted a person's grave illness, but also raised questions about the malleability of a victim's race.[17]

Consequently, as the epidemic spread throughout August, many New Orleanians became terrified to venture from their homes, which they still considered to be relatively safe private spaces. The healthy hoped to avoid exposure to miasmas in public, and the sick, particularly if they were jaundiced, worried about their standing in the community and therefore often preferred to convalesce or die alone. As a result, many undiscovered corpses rotted in private until the odor of decay alerted wary neighbors to a victim's presence. Then, in a misguided and apparently fruitless effort to mask the cloying smell of death and rid New Orleans of dangerous vapors, the city government only fouled the environment further when it began burning barrels of tar at major intersections. As thick, greasy smoke wafted through the already polluted air, many more people avoided the outdoors, leaving most of the city's public spaces, including the streets, "deserted." With the entire city at a standstill, terrified New Orleanians scanned the papers for death notices, cared for the sick, and prayed that the epidemic might spare them for another day. A. J. Wood, an architect working in the city during the outbreak, wrote: "the faculties are stunned and awed, the senses are oppressed with the deepest gloom. Never have I known such cause for sadness." Another depressed observer, summing up the state of affairs, noted that by the middle of the month, "the whole city was a hospital."[18]

This assessment sheds light on conditions in New Orleans in August 1853: death, normally private and sacred, had become public and all too commonplace, as the city grappled with the transformative power of disease, the frailty of white bodies, and the horror of mass mortality. In early August, with countless vectors carrying the yellow fever pathogen throughout New Orleans, and thousands of people hosting the virus, the epidemic had statistical probability on its side, as the likelihood of a mosquito spreading the disease from one person to the next reached its apex. The results were terrifying, even by the standards of 1853. On 1 August, the *Daily Delta* reported that nearly seven hundred people had died from yellow fever the previous week. The next week that number jumped to over one thousand and stayed at least that high for the next month. New Orleanians read the signs of such carnage all around them. As the daily death toll exceeded two hundred in the third week of August, "every awning post" on the city's once busy streets was "placarded with funeral invitations," leaving the few remaining pedestrians "melancholy" as they "noticed the names of the dead." Somber processions, looking like parades gone horribly wrong, carried hundreds of bodies through the gates of New Orleans's cemeteries. Death had become ubiquitous in the city.[19]

In this horrifying setting, although New Orleanians had no idea that yellow fever was contagious, or that mosquitoes served as the virus's vector, they did understand that a plot for a slave uprising could spread through the city like fire. Whereas mounting a rebellion in the rural South presented nearly insurmountable obstacles—organizing resistance across great distances between plantations was next to impossible—in an urban environment the task was far simpler. The way crowd diseases circulate in cities provides a fair analogy, albeit anachronistic because of the limits of medical knowledge at the time: word of a slave conspiracy could grow geometrically, as each carrier might share knowledge with several other people. The problem for white New Orleanians, already anxious about race and yellow fever, thus became more dire, as a huge free community of color lived side by side with slaves in the city, and many light-skinned African Americans were able to pass for white if they wished. That New Orleans's waterfront was among the world's busiest ports made the situation still more frightening, as transients of all races and ethnicities constantly traveled through town, making supervision of local people of color a formidable task. All of which helps explains why, as yellow fever began killing hundreds of white New Orleanians daily in mid-August 1853, the city's supposedly immune *gens de couleur libres* and slaves could seem as threatening as the epidemic.[20]

By the middle of August, the only crowded places in New Orleans, besides hospitals, were cemeteries, so-called cities of the dead. Because much of the city lies below sea level and sits atop a high water table, underground burials were mostly impracticable until the turn of the twentieth century. Accordingly, most of New Orleans's oldest cemeteries are made up of a series of elaborate crypts and tombs where wealthier residents are laid to rest, and row upon row of multitiered vaults, similar to the lockers of a morgue, which are the final resting place for the less affluent. In the summer of 1853, though, there were too few vaults and crypts available for the epidemic's victims, so corpses were often buried in an effort to limit the production of miasmas. Unfortunately, as the number of victims climbed each day in August, the city's cemeteries started overflowing, bringing mass death into plain view.

As New Orleanians faced the widespread spectacle of death and its postmortem impact in 1853, white bodies became even more public. The Fourth District Cemetery hosted some of the most horrific and oft-discussed calamities. On Friday, 4 August, workers lugged seventy-one corpses to the Fourth District, where six men struggled to keep pace interring bodies. Overwhelmed, the workers finally gave up, leaving forty coffins sitting out in the heat—daytime highs were in the nineties—and humidity over the weekend. In a scathing exposé, a journalist reported, "the action of the sun, through the frail enclosures, produced a rapid decomposition of the bodies, several of which swelled so as to burst the coffins." The smell of decay, an "unusually violent and offensive effluvia," drew people from the surrounding neighborhood to the site of the charnel, and the horrified onlookers reported the awful scene to municipal authorities. In another gruesome instance, the city's climate, geology, and topography intersected to make more mayhem, as rushed and weary laborers buried scores of coffins beneath only a light sprinkling of soil, "in the manner of potato ridges." With the first heavy rains they floated back above ground, funereal rafts navigating the city's streets.[21]

Repelled yet apparently fascinated by these spectacles of public death and mortification, editors at the *Daily Delta* took "a visit to the cemetery" and reported their findings in lurid fashion worthy of the dime novels of the day. As the *Delta's* writers entered the graveyard, they were appalled to see "several little children engaged in the most joyous merriment, and an old woman vending ice cream to passers-by, who had to hold camphor to their noses to avoid fainting from the odor." The authors then employed a vast array of adjectives, recounting rows of coffins, clouds of flies circling them, and foul odors in the air. Two days later, a voyeur on the *Daily Crescent* staff outdid his colleague at the *Delta* for macabre detail. In the *Crescent's* story, the sinister gravediggers made "haste with another morsel contributed to the grand banquet of death"; the lone woman by the gates had multiplied into groups of "old and withered crones and fat huckster women, fretting in their own grease, dispensing ice creams and confection"; and the insects had transformed into swarms of "green bottle-flies that hovered on their merchandise, and that anon buzzed away to drink dainty inhalations from the green and festering corpses." The decomposition of white bodies had become a public spectacle.[22]

Beyond a ghoulish, and perhaps, given the circumstances, understandable fascination with bodily corruption, the stories' implications were clear: the epidemic had sullied one of the city's most sacred rituals. This theme was expressed in a detail both papers included in their articles. Due to a shortage of able-bodied white men, it seems that New Orleans's government, confronted with the prospect of a series of disasters similar to the one taking place at the Fourth District Cemetery, turned to African-American slaves and free people of color to dig graves. The city first deployed convict labor—chain gangs of slaves—to cemeteries requiring assistance. When the epidemic drained that pool of free labor, officials offered the huge sum of five dollars per hour, as well as food and drink, including alcoholic beverages dispensed graveside, for service hauling coffins and interring bodies. Then, in the week leading to 14 August, as more than fifteen hundred people died from yellow fever, still more African Americans were impressed into the ranks of the gravediggers, while others willingly seized the chance to make relatively large sums of quick cash.[23]

Under normal circumstances, gravediggers typically—and often, in service of decorum, intentionally—fall into a vast realm of hidden laborers, people whose work goes unnoticed much of the time. During the epidemic of 1853, though, these jobs and the people doing them were subject to intense scrutiny in New Orleans. In part this was so because death and its attendant rites became a matter of open discourse during the yellow fever outbreak. The intense demand for gravediggers and the grim debacles that resulted from the labor shortage also contributed to popular fascination with these workers and their task. Racial anxiety, though, was a more important factor in spurring the public debates. Funerals in New Orleans were holy events, sanctified and usually segregated rituals that remained private even as they took place in public space. The sight of healthy African Americans burying dead white bodies, including corpses of elite Creoles and individuals thought to have acclimated to the local environs, thus discomfited many New Orleanians, as it proved that yellow fever had overturned even the city's most durable racial hierarchies, not to mention long-standing medical misconceptions.[24]

Hushed worries about the phantom slave insurrection increased popular anxiety about African-American gravediggers. Still more troubling, people of color were not succumbing to yellow fever (public health workers later estimated that fewer than 150 African Americans had died from yellow fever during the summer of 1853). The presence of unfamiliar African Americans crossing the color line at funerals, therefore, seemed not only profane, but also threatening, as black bodies apparently remained untouched by illness even during the epidemic's darkest days, while whites succumbed in ever greater numbers. Some white mourners found their racial anxieties embodied in the image of African-Americans laboring in cemeteries without shirts, a concession that overseers allowed due to the brutal summer heat. A reporter literally on the graveyard shift at the *Daily Delta* recounted the presence of "half naked negroes" lugging caskets and interring corpses, menacing images for white onlookers who hoped to bury their departed loved ones without being confronted by the robust bodies of the city's people of color.[25]

Although the papers grudgingly admitted that the African-American laborers "who superintended the burials, observed a proper solemnity and performed their disagreeable duties in a becoming manner," many New Orleanians remained upset by the breakdown in social and spatial segregation at gravesites. This was yet another example of the way the epidemic had upended normal life in the city, these frustrated observers suggested. After all, by August 1853, the epidemic had become so terrible that whites could not even attend to their own dead. Ultimately, though, few people had any choice in the matter. Either African Americans would be allowed—even encouraged—to bury white bodies for high pay, or corpses would continue to decay in plain view, above ground, further desecrating the dead, spawning more miasmas, and generating additional anxiety in the city. Eventually, many New Orleanians apparently reconciled themselves to this shocking turn of events by acknowledging that digging graves was depressing, taxing, and (supposedly) dangerous. And thus, most onlookers finally agreed, it was inhuman work ideally suited to African Americans who were often thrust into jobs that whites found abhorrent in the city, throughout the South, and nationwide.[26]

In part, expediency and the South's social and racial caste system explain why New Orleanians finally accepted African Americans digging graves during the epidemic. But reputed African-American immunity to yellow fever proved even more compelling for many people, as digging graves seemed a reasonable (and punitive) way to deal with people of color who were not succumbing to disease. Throughout the antebellum era, the South's medical community observed that African Americans rarely contracted yellow fever. Over time, many of the region's physicians began arguing that slaves and *gens de couleur libres* were immune to the disease because of a host of bodily attributes, all ostensibly unique to slaves and free people of color. Dr. Samuel Cartwright, among others, gained fame for studies of the "physical peculiarities of the negro race." Passing over acclimation, Cartwright and his peers posited other sources for African-American immunity, pointing instead to a host of physical, or what they called natural attributes, such as skin pigmentation and an enlarged liver. Cartwright, for instance, wrote, "the difference in the organic or physical characters imprinted by the hand of Nature on the two races" accounted for African-American immunity. Other physicians concurred, arguing that slaves and free people of color were "naturally" immune to the disease, because of both observable corporeal traits and their continent of origin.[27]

In 1853, these pseudoscientific studies of African-American bodies offered one way for some New Orleanians to cope with their racial anxiety. While New Orleans's Creoles proudly wore their reputed immunity to yellow fever as a badge of honor, African-American resistance to the disease carried social stigma. Because of the theory of acclimation, immunity among Creoles represented permanence in New Orleans. For whites generally, immunity and good health connoted social standing, while New Orleanians typically viewed susceptibility to disease as symptomatic of impurity, transience, and poverty. For slaves and free people of color, though, immunity symbolized ties to the untamed and uncivilized nature found on the "dark continent" of Africa, as well as bodily difference. Cartwright and his colleagues therefore insisted that slaves' and free people of color's "primitive" condition insulated them from disease; that they emitted odd odors which repelled sickness; and that they sweated copiously, flushing yellow fever from their bodies even if they somehow contracted the disease. Extrapolating wildly, these physicians argued that African Americans were "perfect non-conductors of yellow fever," going so far as to suggest that during the summer months, New Orleans should array a phalanx of slaves along its riverfront, a human levee designed to keep back a flood of pestilence.[28]

As a way of further placating anxious New Orleanians who felt threatened by the sight of healthy African-Americans burying the city's dead, Cartwright and his cohort conscripted nature into what they deemed a holy war, employing their findings as planks (albeit rotten ones) in the proslavery platform. Practicing what one historian has labeled "states' rights medicine," these quacks drew on environmental determinism as a wellspring for their scientific racism, arguing that "nature" had kindly provided white Southerners with an African-American population immune to yellow fever. Facing off with abolitionists who wrote in Northern antislavery papers such as Horace Greeley's *New York Tribune* that the epidemic was the cleansing hand of God, Cartwright sneered and turned such arguments topsy-turvy, noting that "nature scorns to see the aristocracy of the white skin . . . reduced to drudgery under a Southern sun, and has issued her fiat." Capitalizing on the corporeal fears that people had about the origins and racial implications of suntans, Cartwright raged that white men, and recent immigrants to New Orleans particularly, who engaged in menial labor "waged war against Nature by making negroes of themselves in laboring in the sun." Nature, the doctor insisted, intended for white bodies to remain white; those who ignored this biological imperative would reap the whirlwind.[29]

With sectional concerns already a hot topic in New Orleans in the months leading to the epidemic and the phantom slave insurrection, and news of Harriet Beecher Stowe's travels in Europe still plastered across the city's headlines during the outbreak, local slaveholders, many of whom were facing the prospect for the first time that their heritage might not insulate them from illness, likely took particular comfort in Cartwright's theories. Quite soon, editors at the proslavery *Daily Delta,* which catered to the city's Creole elite, joined the chorus of Cartwright's supporters, observing that most of the whites who had succumbed to yellow fever during the epidemic had done "work in the hot noon-day summer's sun, that the negroes ought to do." Embracing a paternalistic argument, the *Delta* claimed, "Negroes who have masters to take care of them, never die with yellow fever. If they do die, it is because they have been practicing the abolition theory." Slavery was not just a necessary evil; it was a positive good. Disloyal slaves, or people of color unlucky enough to be free, were more likely to contract and die from yellow fever. The writer at the *Delta* followed this flawed line of reasoning to its logical dead end, concluding that the epidemic might have been avoided entirely if African Americans had done the city's heavy lifting, as nature intended, leaving whites to work better suited to them.[30]

The question of whether African Americans were or are immune to yellow fever remains unanswered. Many epidemiologists argue that what appears to be inherent immunity is actually a product of high levels of acquired immunity, somehow akin to a process of acclimation. Other experts insist that prolonged exposure to the disease across generations in Africa, where yellow fever was endemic, yielded genetic resistance. If African-American imperviousness to yellow fever is biologically founded, still other scholars suggest, the disease acted as another kind of biological revenge for the slave trade, laying waste to Euro-Americans while African Americans enjoyed genetic resistance to illness. Ironically, though, this revenge only increased Euro-American hunger for slaves by devastating pools of Native and Euro-American workers in the South, thus supporting the contention of scientific racists like Cartwright and his cohort that "nature" had "formed" African Americans to work in the region's heat and humidity by rendering them immune to yellow fever. Still, though this sounds like a recipe for environmental racism—and it sometimes was—at least during the epidemic of 1853, some African Americans took advantage of their alleged and apparent immunity, challenging New Orleans's social and spatial order as they worked for relatively high pay in public.[31]

"THE NECROPOLIS OF THE SOUTH"

Although many New Orleanians believed that the epidemic had to have reached its zenith with the horrors at the Fourth District Cemetery, the death toll rose still higher throughout August. More than fifteen hundred people were dying weekly by the middle of the month, and the twenty-first became known as the "black day," when approximately three hundred people succumbed to yellow fever. With the "city almost wholly at a stand," and public landscapes empty, morale sank to new depths, and New Orleanians looked to the heavens as they grappled with their frailties. In the month's last week, each of the city's major religious denominations sponsored public prayer meetings. Collectively, supplicants sank to their knees before a God they hoped would be merciful, acknowledging that they had "grievously sinned." Mayor Crossman tried to use the city's pious mood to his advantage when he cast the pestilence not as a failure of government, but as an act of God. He set aside 2 September as a day of fasting and prayer, during which people would "close their stores, offices, shops and public places" in order to placate the "Supreme Being" who had chosen "to lay the heavy hand of Pestilence on" New Orleans. As one cleric suggested when he wrote to the archbishop of New Orleans, "the science of the doctors is powerless against God." The epidemic had undermined people's faith in human agency when compared to the terrible power of the nonhuman world.[32]

Following the public prayers, the weekly death toll began declining. Some New Orleanians believed that their pleas had been answered by a kindly deity, but it is more likely that the outbreak receded for epidemiological and environmental reasons. Based on the number of deaths reported in the city by mid-September, yellow fever had killed at least eight thousand people during the summer of 1853. Even assuming a remarkably high ratio of deaths to recoveries, it is likely that at least sixteen thousand more people had contracted and survived the virus during the epidemic, leaving those individuals immune to future attacks. After accounting for the vast horde of migrants who fled the city—one source guessed that only seventy-five thousand people, or about half of New Orleans's regular population, had remained through the summer—and the portion of the city's population that had acquired immunity during previous epidemics, it is fair to conclude that by September the available reservoir of hosts for yellow fever had begun evaporating. With autumn's approach, the virus's vector, too, began disappearing. In mid-September, temperatures in the city fell into the fifties, and the cooler weather limited the remaining mosquitoes' efficiency as disease couriers. The result was fewer than one thousand deaths for the month: a fearful total in past epidemics, but cause for celebration in 1853.[33]

In September's second week, when only four hundred people died from yellow fever, many New Orleanians considered how the city might best recover from the epidemic and the rumored slave insurrection. The first order of business for the commercial community was rehabilitating New Orleans's battered public image, a process that yielded a number of wild claims, including shrill denials that pestilence had struck the city hard and further hollow assertions about the benevolence of local slaveholders. As historian Conevery Bolton Valencius argues, locations can become associated with illness, a damaging reputation that lingers long after an epidemic's end. Even prior to 1853, wary onlookers had called New Orleans a "wet graveyard," "the necropolis of the South," or, as one tourist put it after visiting the city, "the head-quarters of Death." Many local businesspeople believed that these perceptions had limited New Orleans's economic growth. As a result, the city's commercial community had tried to spread the word that yellow fever had released its grip on New Orleans. Even while admitting that the city was "sometimes overtaken with epidemics," these boosters had insisted that New Orleans did "not suffer in a fair and liberal comparison, in respect to public health, with many others reputed to be more healthy."[34]

Over time, projecting the image that New Orleans was healthy had become a matter of civic duty. Admitting that yellow fever had returned to the city, therefore, struck a blow against commerce, against growth, and against progress. In the epidemic's aftermath, Dr. Morton Dowler noted that "commerce is King and it is no more permitted to any physician to report cases of fever . . . than to foretell and encompass the King's death." Dowler also raged that "the influences exist, in this city, which prevent the actual state of public health, during the summer months, so far as yellow fever is concerned, from being known to the people." Although nearly ten thousand fatalities from yellow fever certainly complicated ongoing efforts at maintaining an official silence, they did not entirely stop them. In the autumn of 1853, New Orleans's papers published a steady stream of stories suggesting that "all signs of the late pestilence have been obliterated," and that "there is scarcely a visible mark or scar left by the epidemic." Even after a cholera outbreak killed more than six hundred people late in the fall, the press still claimed that "no prudent or temperate person need entertain any doubt but that at the present time he can abide in New Orleans as safely and healthily as anywhere in the Union."[35]

The press used similar rhetoric in its efforts to quiet lingering discussions about rebellious slaves in the city. As soon as the morning after George Wright spoke to Chief O'Leary, many businesspeople and the editors who relied on them for advertising revenue had tried to keep talk of the insurrection quiet. As with word of yellow fever, though, news of racial violence traveled quickly and threatened commerce as it made its way up the Mississippi. To counter such developments, the city papers promised, "there is nothing in history to equal the peaceable submission of the African slaves to the paternal government of the whites in the Southern States of this Union." The rebellion, the press insisted, was a farce. Still, the chatter had echoed through the summer, and with the epidemic's end, the *Daily Picayune* redoubled its efforts, excoriating London's papers for pandering to British abolitionists with a series about the fear of insurrection that was gripping New Orleans. The *Daily Delta* went further, clinging to the idea that slavery accounted for a low mortality rate among the city's people of color: "we refer to the conclusion in favor of slavery, deducible from the exemption of our blacks from the attacks of a fever which seizes nineteen-twentieths of our white population." Creole immunity and acclimation might have faltered, but at least kindly masters had kept their slaves safe, the *Delta* suggested. New Orleans thus had nothing to fear from chattel slaves, grateful to their owners for protection from illness. In this regard, at least, little had changed in the city.[36]

Still, in 1853, racial anxiety spawned a rebellion in New Orleans, a phantom slave insurrection that terrified many of the city's residents for six months. Worries about disloyal slaves had less to do with the particulars of a foiled plot or the long odds of its success and more to do with the nature of urban ecology and the transformative properties of epidemic illness. That yellow fever attacked white New Orleanians who counted themselves immune to disease overturned enduring assumptions in the city about urban spaces, ethnicity, and class privilege. That the virus then turned white New Orleanians into people of color, if only briefly, while sparing slaves and *gens de couleur libres,* played into popular fears about the plasticity of racial identity and the city's social castes. Bodies of all kinds, usually the most private of spaces, could host organisms that moved throughout New Orleans from one person and place to the next without regard for issues of class, cultural heritage, or cleanliness. People, New Orleanians learned to their horror, could become public spaces, their bodies as subject to reworking, contestation, and negotiation as a community park, marketplace, or waterfront.

NOTES

1. *New Orleans Daily Delta,* 15, 16 June 1853; *New Orleans Daily Picayune,* 14 June 1853.

2. Quote from *New Orleans Daily Picayune,* 14 June 1853. See also: *New Orleans Daily Delta,* 14 June 1853; *New Orleans Weekly Delta,* 19 June 1853.

3. Quote from *New Orleans Daily Picayune,* 16 June 1853. See also: L. H. Webb Diaries, entry for 14 June 1853, in Louisiana State Museum, Record Group 49; New Orleans Office of the Mayor, Letter Books, 1811–1920, entries for 14 June 1853, in New Orleans Public Library, New Orleans City Archives Collection, Record Group AA 511.

4. Quotes from *New Orleans Daily Picayune,* 19 June 1853; ibid., 16 June 1853; L. H. Webb Diaries, entry for 14 June 1853; *New Orleans Daily Picayune,* 19 June 1853.

5. Quote from *New Orleans Daily Picayune,* 19 June 1853. See also: John Blasingame, *Black New Orleans* (Chicago: University of Chicago Press, 1973), pp. 1, 9; *New Orleans Daily Delta,* 14–18, 20, 22 June 1853; *New Orleans Daily Picayune,* 14–16, 18, 22, 25 June 1853; *New Orleans Weekly Delta,* 19 June 1853; New Orleans Office of the Mayor, Letter Books, 1811–1920, entries for 14, 16, 22, 29 June 1853, in New Orleans Public Library, New Orleans City Archives Collection, Record Group AA 511; Robert C. Reinders, *End of an Era: New Orleans, 1850–1860* (New Orleans: Pelican Publishing, 1964), p. 23.

6. John Duffy, *Sword of Pestilence* (Baton Rouge: Louisiana State University Press, 1966), p. vii.

7. Quote from *Report of the Sanitary Commission of New Orleans on the Yellow Fever Epidemic of 1853* (New Orleans: Picayune Office, 1854), p. 22. See also: "Health, Mortality, Etc.," *New Orleans Medical and Surgical Journal* 10 (September 1853): 275.

8. *New Orleans Daily Picayune,* 19, 21, 23 June 1853; B. Dowler, "On the Necropolis of New Orleans," *New Orleans Medical and Surgical Journal* 7 (November 1850): 277; M. Morton Dowler, "On the Reported Causes of Yellow Fever and the So Called Sanitary Measures of the Day," ibid., 11 (July 1854): 44; *New Orleans Daily Delta,* 6 October 1853; *New Orleans Daily Crescent,* 22 June 1853; "History and Incidents of the Plague in New Orleans," *Harpers* 7 (November 1853): 797; E. D. Fenner, *History of the Epidemic Yellow Fever at New Orleans, La., in 1853* (New York: Hall, Clayton, & Co., Printers, 1854), p. 4; New Orleans Office of the Mayor, Letter Books, 1811–1920, entries for June 1–7, 1853, in New Orleans Public Library, New Orleans City Archives Collection, Record Group AA 511.

9. Jo Ann Carrigan, *Saffron Scourge* (Lafayette, La.: Center for Louisiana Studies, 1994), pp. 33, 55; Margaret Humphreys, *Yellow Fever and the South* (New Brunswick,

N.J.: Rutgers University Press, 1992), pp. 3–23; Charles Rosenberg, *Explaining Epidemics* (Cambridge: Cambridge University Press, 1992), p. 297.

10. Quote from *New Orleans Daily Delta,* 22 July 1853. See also: Samuel A. Cartwright, "Review of the Meteorology, Vital Statistics, and Hygiene of the State of Louisiana," *New Orleans Medical Society Journal* 8 (September 1851): 238–49; Suzanne E. Hatty and James Hatty, *The Disordered Body* (Albany: State University of New York Press, 1999), p. 43; K. David Patterson, "Yellow Fever Epidemics and Mortality in the United States, 1693–1905," *Social Science and Medicine* 34 (1992): 863; Joseph E. Tregle, Jr., "Creoles and Americans," in *Creole New Orleans,* ed. Arnold R. Hirsch and Joseph Logsdon (Baton Rouge: Louisiana State University Press, 1992), p. 135.

11. Patterson, "Yellow Fever Epidemics and Mortality in the United States, 1693–1905," p. 863.

12. Quotes from *New Orleans Daily Picayune,* 30 July 1853; George Washington Cable, *The Creoles of Louisiana* (New York: Charles Scribner's Sons, 1884), p. 292. See also: John Higham, *Strangers in the Land* (New Brunswick, N.J.: Rutgers University Press, 1955), pp. 5–13; Judith Walzer Leavitt, *Typhoid Mary* (New York: Beacon Press, 1997), pp. 11–32.

13. Quotes from "Health, Mortality, Etc.," *New Orleans Medical and Surgical Journal* 10 (September 1853): 275; *New Orleans Daily Delta,* 25 July 1853; Zachary Robertson to Decius Beebe, 27 July 1853, Beebe Family Papers, Louisiana State Museum Historical Center, Record Group 46. See also *New Orleans Daily Delta,* 1 August 1853.

14. Quotes from Patterson, "Yellow Fever Epidemics and Mortality in the United States, 1693–1905," p. 863; *Report of the Sanitary Commission of New Orleans on the Yellow Fever Epidemic of 1853,* p. 354. See also: A. N. Clements, *The Physiology of Mosquitoes* (New York: Macmillan, 1963), p. 302; Jack C. Jones, "The Feeding Behavior of Mosquitoes," *Scientific American,* no. 238 (June 1978): 138; Lawrence Lacey and Bruce Orr, "The Role of Biological Control of Mosquitoes in Integrated Vector Control," *American Journal of Tropical Medicine and Hygiene* 50, suppl. (1994): 107; P. F. Mattingly, *The Biology of Mosquito-Borne Disease* (London: George Allen and Unwin, 1969), pp. 21–24; Jean Slosek, "Aedes Aegypti Mosquitoes in the Americas: A Review of Their Interactions with the Human Population," *Social Science Medicine* 23 (1986): 252.

15. Quotes from L. H. Webb Diaries, 1, 6 June 1853; *New Orleans Daily Delta,* 29 June 1853. See also ibid., 16 June 1853.

16. *New Orleans Daily Picayune,* 30 July 1853; *New Orleans Bee,* 29 July 1853.

17. Coneverey Bolton Valencius, *The Health of the Country* (New York: Basic Books, 2002), pp. 1–14, 53–84; Jennifer Michel Spear, "'Whiteness and the Purity of Blood': Race, Sexuality, and Social Order in Colonial Louisiana" (Ph.D. diss., University of Minnesota, 1999), pp. 1–54, 101–54, 195–224.

18. Quotes from William Robinson, *Diary of a Samaritan* (New York: Harper and Brothers, 1860), p. 161; Thomas Keelah Wharton Diary, entry for 22 August 1853, in Manuscripts and Rare Books Division, New York Public Library; Robinson, *Diary of a Samaritan,* p. 150.

19. Quotes from Zachary Robertson to Decius Beebe, 27 July 1853, Beebe Family Papers, Louisiana State Museum Historical Center, Record Group 46. See also *New Orleans Daily Delta,* 1, 8 August 1853.

20. Ari Kelman, *A River and Its City: The Nature of Landscape in New Orleans* (Berkeley: University of California Press, 2003), pp. 50–154.

21. Quotes from *New Orleans Daily Delta,* 8 August 1853; "The Plague in the Southwest," *De Bow's Review of the Southern and Western States,* n.s. 15, no. 1 (December 1853): 619.

22. Quotes from *New Orleans Daily Delta,* 9 August 1853; *New Orleans Daily Crescent,* 11 August 1853.

23. *New Orleans Daily Delta,* 9 August 1853; Fenner, *History of the Epidemic Yellow Fever,* p. 38.

24. Fenner, *History of the Epidemic Yellow Fever,* p. 38; *New Orleans Daily Delta,* 9 August, 1 September 1853; *New Orleans Daily Picayune,* 28 August 1853.

25. Quote from *New Orleans Daily Delta,* 1 September 1853. See also *New Orleans Daily Picayune,* 4, 11–13, 17, 24, 28 August 1853.

26. Quote from *New Orleans Daily Delta,* 1 September 1853. See also Blasingame, *Black New Orleans,* pp. 1–27.

27. Quotes from Samuel A. Cartwright, "Report on the Diseases and Physical Peculiarities of the Negro Race," *New Orleans Medical and Surgical Journal* 7 (May 1851): 201 and 187 respectively; A. Hester, M.D., "Medical History of Two Epidemic Yellow Fevers," *New Orleans Medical and Surgical Journal* 7 (July 1850): 82; and J. C. Nott, "The Epidemic of Yellow Fever in Mobile in 1853," ibid., 10 (March 1854): 577.

28. Quotes from Hester, "Medical History of Two Epidemic Yellow Fevers," p. 82; Samuel A. Cartwright, "Prevention of Yellow Fever," *New Orleans Medical and Surgical Journal* 10 (November 1853): 316.

29. Quotes from Marie Louise Marshall, "Samuel A. Cartwright and States' Rights Medicine," *New Orleans Medical and Surgical Journal* 93 (August 1940): 75; Cartwright, "Prevention of Yellow Fever," p. 312; Cartwright, "Review of the Meteorology, Vital Statistics, and Hygiene of the State of Louisiana," p. 246. See also: *New Orleans Daily Delta,* 23 September 1853; *New Orleans Daily Picayune,* 29 September 1853.

30. Quotes from *New Orleans Daily Delta,* 14 August 1853. See also ibid., 5, 23 June, 28 July, 15 September 1853.

31. Quote from Hester, "Medical History of Two Epidemic Yellow Fevers," p. 82. See also: Kenneth F. Kiple and Virginia H. Kiple, "Black Yellow Fever Immunities, Innate and Acquired, as Revealed in the American South," *Social Science History* 1 (Summer 1977): 420; K. David Patterson, "Disease Environments of the Antebellum South," in *Science and Medicine in the Old South,* ed. Ronald L. Numbers and Todd Savitt (Baton Rouge: Louisiana State University Press, 1989), p. 164.

32. Quotes from *New Orleans Daily Delta,* 23 August 1853; *New Orleans Price Current and Daily Intelligencer,* 27 August 1853; *New Orleans Daily Picayune,* 24 August 1853; Proclamation of the Mayoralty of New Orleans, 30 August 1853, in New Orleans Office of the Mayor, Letter Books 1811–1920, New Orleans Public Library, New Orleans City Archives Collection; Edward E. Legendre to Archbishop Anthony Blanc, 11 August 1853, in Correspondence Collection, Archives of the Archdiocese of New Orleans. See also: Fenner, *History of the Epidemic Yellow Fever at New Orleans,* p. 38; Ted Steinberg, *Acts of God* (Oxford: Oxford University Press, 2000), p. 19.

33. "Meteorological Register for New Orleans," in *Report of the Sanitary Commission of New Orleans on the Yellow Fever Epidemic of 1853,* unpaginated table; *New Orleans Daily Crescent,* 26 September 1853; *New Orleans Daily Delta,* 1 October 1853.

34. Quotes from B. Dowler, "On the Necropolis of New Orleans," *New Orleans Medical and Surgical Journal* 7 (November 1850): 277; Henry Tudor, *Narrative of a Tour of North America,* vol. 2 (London: James Duncan, 1834), p. 64; "Health of the City," *New Orleans Medical and Surgical Journal* 8 (July 1851): 135. See also: Conevery Bolton Valencius, "The Geography of Health and the Making of the American West," in *Medical Geography in Historical Perspective,* ed. Nicolaas Rupke (London: The Wellcome Trust Centre for the History of Medicine at UCL, 2000), pp. 122–27; *New Orleans Bee,* 19 September 1853.

35. Quotes from M. Morton Dowler, "On the Reported Causes of Yellow Fever and the So Called Sanitary Measures of the Day," p. 44; *New Orleans Daily Delta,* 6 October, 26 November, 25 November 1853.

36. Quotes from *New Orleans Weekly Delta,* 19 June, 23 September 1853. See also *New Orleans Daily Picayune,* 29 September 1853.

2

Green Space and Class in Imperial London

Peter Thorsheim

Well-to-do people, unless they personally interest themselves in the welfare of the industrial and poorer classes, can form no adequate conception of the sad condition . . . under which tens of thousands of them live and die. Unless in the neighbourhood of a park—and but a very small proportion of the labouring class reside within easy reach of such open spaces—the only opportunity they have of relaxation and recreation is in the busy thoroughfares, while their children for the most part have no playground but the gutter and the pavement.

—*The Times* (London), 11 September 1884

On 5 May 1884 a group of eminent Victorians made their way to one of the least auspicious places in London. Traveling south of the River Thames through the predominantly working-class borough of Southwark, they ended their journey at a partially demolished prison known as the Horsemonger Lane Gaol. It was here, eight decades earlier, that the Irish conspirator Edward Despard and six of his accomplices had been publicly hanged, disemboweled, and beheaded. Their purpose on this day was not to commemorate these executions, however, but to preside over a public ceremony that marked the conversion of the site to an altogether different purpose.

The proceedings opened on a festive note, with a police marching band performing selections from the *William Tell* overture and *H.M.S. Pinafore,* along with the inevitable "God Save the Queen." Among the dignitaries in attendance were Catherine Gladstone (the prime minister's wife), Sir Robert Peel (son of the statesman who had established the Metropolitan Police and thereby inspired the term "bobbies"), and Lord Aberdeen (who later served as viceroy of Ireland). The presence of so distinguished a group at this dedication played a vital role in helping to transform its setting from a place associated with crime and brutality to one of respectability and wholesome activity. In his speech marking the occasion, Peel expressed his hope "that the place which had witnessed so much sorrow would be one of happiness to many generations of children." Henceforth, it would be a playground.[1]

The new playground was an immediate sensation. During the first summer it was open, an average of two thousand children visited it each day. In it they were able to run, play games, and exercise using gymnastic equipment donated by the Metropolitan Public Gardens Association, a group established in 1882 by the Anglo-Irish aristocrat Reginald Brabazon.[2] In the years that followed, he and his allies sought to build on their success by preserving and opening green spaces throughout the British capital. In doing so, they unleashed a torrent of debate about property rights, respectability, and degeneration in imperial London.

Property

Accessible green space was extremely limited in many parts of Victorian London. Already home to a million people in 1800, the metropolis expanded rapidly in both area and population during the nineteenth century. By 1900 well over six million people lived in the conurbation that was Greater London.[3] This process entailed enormous changes in land use at the city's expanding periphery as previously rural places became urban. No less important, however, were the ways in which population growth, along with expanding commerce and new technology, changed the character of places that had long been part of the metropolis. The construction of houses, offices, warehouses, and railway stations placed great demands on urban space and caused property values to rise sharply. As this happened, many came to view London's geography as a physical manifestation of class difference. Unlike Britain's other cities, which were small enough to be escaped easily on foot, London's size meant that many of its inhabitants rarely saw the countryside. Although London contained nine public parks at mid-century, only one—Victoria Park—was situated in the East End. In the decades of enormous growth that followed, the disparity continued. Within a four-mile radius of Charing Cross, according to an analysis published in the 1880s, the western half of London contained eight times as many acres of parks and gardens as did the eastern half.[4] In the words of one observer, although London had "undergone a wonderful transformation" in recent decades, "its inhabitants, especially the poorer classes, suffer in consequence."[5]

Attention to these changes grew in the late nineteenth century as London came to be seen as an "imperial metropolis."[6] Reflecting this perspective, the best-selling novelist and essayist Ouida (Marie Louise de la Ramée) suggested in 1888 that judicious planning, rather than laissez-faire property development, was necessary to create an urban landscape worthy of London's imperial role: "For a city which is in some respects the greatest capital of the world, the approaches to London are of singular and painful unsightliness. What can the Indian prince, the Asiatic monarch, the Continental ambassador, or the Oriental envoy, think when his first acquaintance with it is made in the confusion and hideousness of Cannon Street, or in the disorder and nakedness of Charing Cross Station?"[7] In her estimation, Londoners suffered from insufficient contact with nature largely because the rich refused to share it. "When the beauty and wealth of a great society are displayed in its architecture, in its gardens, in its public pageantries and festivals, then the body of the public is a sharer in and gainer by them; what is left of beauty in London is wholly shut away behind the iron gates of courtyards and the hall doors of noble mansions."[8] Too much, in other words, had been left in the hands of private individuals who devoted more attention to profits than to aesthetic form, urban function, or the public good.

Even for Londoners who were fortunate enough to live near green space, proximity was no guarantee of access or unhampered use. During the seventeenth and eighteenth centuries, middle- and upper-class residents built tall fences and installed locked gates around squares; only those who owned the fashionable houses that surrounded them possessed the keys.[9] As a result, working-class children frequently lacked any place other than the street in which to play. During a single summer's day in 1890, three children died after being run over by horse-drawn vehicles near King's Cross railway station. The neighborhood contained several squares and small gardens, but none of them allowed children to play in them.[10] To compensate for the lack of accessible green space in London, reformers came up with a variety of novel proposals. Some suggested creating subterranean playgrounds, while others recommended establishing them on rooftops. While the latter proposal afforded the promise of being outdoors, the quality of the air at roof level was far from ideal. At least one rooftop playground was reportedly built in London, but it was forced to close after only a short time in operation "owing to the extremely sooty appearance which the children bore after a little recreation among the chimneypots."[11]

A letter to the editor of the *Daily News* in 1884, signed "One Who Lives in a Square," decried the "crying sin that so much ground is taken away from the poor in London" by private squares that were closed to all but those who owned the houses that surrounded them. "What a blessing it would be for the poor . . . to be able to send their little children round the corner to play under the trees, when it would be impossible to send them as far off as the park alone."[12] *Reynolds's Newspaper,* a radical daily, similarly condemned "the intolerable meanness of the shopkeepers and others around Lincoln's-inn-fields, who . . . could not think of allowing the offspring of the workers to mingle with their middle-class brats" in its garden. Even when those who "infest[ed] the square" were away on seaside holidays, the gates of the garden remained locked to the poor.[13] In July 1888, the owners of Lincoln's Inn Fields consented to open its seven-acre garden to the public for ninety minutes each evening.[14] The London County Council purchased this land in

1894, creating a public recreation ground. Like the playground that the Metropolitan Public Gardens Association had established at Horsemonger Lane, Lincoln's Inn also had a bloodstained past. A brass marker in the middle of its garden commemorated the supposed spot where William, Lord Russell had been beheaded in 1683 for his alleged involvement in a conspiracy to assassinate King Charles II and his brother, the future James II.[15]

Many property owners protested vehemently against suggestions that they share their squares with nonresidents. In a letter published in 1884, one writer complained that the "insane desire to confer every mortal blessing under the sun on the poor evinced by those who have no boon to confer borders on the ludicrous." He went on to suggest that "to satisfy the irresponsible and democratic tendency of the day," the wealthy might soon be required to allow the poor to live in their drawing rooms. It was just as ridiculous, he maintained, to make London's "peaceful squares . . . the rendezvous and playgrounds of the tag-rag and bob-tail of the streets."[16] In any case, suggested other property owners, it was not necessary to admit poor people to a square for them to derive benefit from it, for its "air spaces and oxygen-exhaling trees" purified an area far beyond its boundary.[17]

Advocates of public parks, gardens, and playgrounds not only put pressure on the owners of green space to grant others access to their property, but also lobbied local government officials to buy private land and dedicate it to public enjoyment. In the 1850s the Hampstead vestry urged the newly formed Metropolitan Board of Works to purchase 200 acres of Hampstead Heath for £50,000, but the board put off a decision because it wanted the central government to contribute at least some of the funds required. Finally, in 1870, 240 acres of Hampstead Heath were purchased for £295,500, a third of which came from subscribers and charity groups.[18] When a nearby piece of land known as Parliament Hill became available in 1885, a committee was formed to ensure that it would not be acquired by builders. Led by the Duke of Westminster, whose family owned large parts of London, and George John Shaw-Lefevre, a Liberal M.P. who led the Commons Preservation Society, the group organized a garden party on the site to convince influential and wealthy Londoners to support their efforts. After a difficult fund-raising campaign that lasted many months, they succeeded in acquiring the land for the public at a cost of £302,000. The Metropolitan Board of Works provided half of the funds, with the rest supplied by individual subscribers, the City of London Charities, and the vestries of St. Pancras, Hampstead, and Marylebone.[19] Applauding the conclusion of the campaign to save this land for the public, the *Graphic* asserted that its importance would "be more and more appreciated as London stretches out its brick-and-mortar battalions further and further into the green fields."[20] At the turn of the twentieth century, according to a contemporary estimate, over a hundred thousand Londoners visited Hampstead's green spaces on a typical bank holiday.[21]

Contact with nature, even in the form of a small garden, was thought helpful in making the lower classes accept the status quo. Octavia Hill, a leading figure in housing reform, smoke abatement, and the National Trust, also played a central role in efforts to preserve green space in cities through a group called the Kyrle Society, which she and her sister Miranda founded in 1877.[22] Hill's vision was liberal, not radical; she vehemently opposed indiscriminate handouts to the poor as well as socialist calls to redistribute wealth. Yet in her view, public access to green space for exercise or recreation was not simply another form of charity, and it was not something that infringed upon private property rights. As Hill put it in 1875, "The house is an individual possession, and should be worked for, but the park or the common which a man shares with his neighbours, which descends as a common inheritance from generation to generation, surely this may be given without pauperising."[23] Interestingly, Hill's ideas about green space and charity echo not only the language that her contemporaries used to promote national parks, but also that of Victorian philanthropists who sought to convert "fallen women" from a life of prostitution to one of moral purity. In 1883, over a decade before she co-founded the National Trust, Hill described the remaining open spaces of London as "wildernesses" that ought to be "rescued" and cared for by an enlightened public body lest they fall "prey" to rapacious and amoral market forces.[24]

PROPRIETY

Destroying Peel's hope that criminality and violence would never return to the site of the former prison at Horsemonger Lane, only a short time after it opened as a place of recreation a twelve-year-old girl was severely beaten while playing in it. So vicious was her assault that her attacker—a sixteen-year-old boy—was sentenced to six months' prison with hard labor.[25] Following this incident, the secretary of the Metropolitan Public Gardens Association rejected the assertions of those who claimed that "the poorer classes were, under the same supervision, more mischievous than those better off."[26] Brabazon's association nonetheless kept a watchful eye on those who visited its gardens and playgrounds. One aspect of this surveillance was its insistence that children who wished to enter the places it controlled be accompanied by someone at least fifteen years old. This requirement may have originated as much from a desire to protect young children from accidents and deliberate harm as from concerns that they would misbehave, but not everyone believed that it was justified. W. F. Baker, a resident of Gray's Inn Road, complained that the group's "obnoxious rule" against unaccompanied children "practically debars the children of poor people from making use of these gardens, as it is absurd to suppose that the poor can employ nursemaids to take their children to these places." Reflecting different assumptions than those of Brabazon's group about the age at which children should assume adult responsibilities, Baker added that it was "nonsense to pretend that children of ten years old and upwards cannot behave themselves properly, more especially as they would know they would be turned out of the garden if they did not do so."[27]

Many middle-class commentators claimed that poor children required not merely adult supervision, but also direction from their social superiors. Writing in a fashionable women's magazine in 1888, Blanche Medhurst claimed that "ladies who volunteer to teach the children games, and to keep order, helping on this true ministering work of humanity, are thus refining and elevating the manners, the ways, the very tones and voices of the children." After just "a few summer weeks of patiently and carefully guided enjoyment of their new playgrounds," children's "roughness tones down," their "wildly excitable shouts and yells are now ringing, happy peals of laughter, and as for the games, there is now awakened in each poor little one that imaginative and receptive power for organised play which makes all natural healthy children what Victor Hugo declared them to be, 'the only true poets.'" As workers gained increasing economic and political power in the late nineteenth century, many of them viewed such paternalism as insulting.[28]

Late Victorian efforts to increase the availability of green space in London occurred during a period of intense anxiety about the human body. In contrast to an earlier age in which capital punishment functioned as a form of popular entertainment and the bodies of the executed were displayed as a warning to others, Victorians became increasingly uncomfortable with such visceral imagery. While the performance of a ballerina or musician was admired because it represented successful discipline and control over the body, the disordered body of someone who was diseased, injured, degenerate, or dead inspired revulsion and fear because it reminded people that no matter how elevated their minds might become, they remained trapped within bodies that were inescapably material.

Although this sensibility also fostered opposition to vivisection and blood sports, its principal focus was human beings. In 1849 a large crowd gathered outside Horsemonger Lane Gaol to witness the double execution of a married couple who had been convicted of murder. The "horror and demoralization" of this event so appalled Charles Dickens that he immediately wrote a letter to the *Times* in which he called for an end to the "ghastly spectacle" of public execution.[29] As a result of the pressure that he and others exerted, the practice was abolished two decades later. Capital punishment continued in Britain for nearly another century, but henceforth it occurred exclusively behind prison walls.

Executions and other forms of physical violence were not the only bodily reminders that reformers sought to banish from public view in Victorian

Britain. Anxieties about the body also contributed to an upsurge in efforts to prevent indecency—making public that which reformers insisted should remain private. This encompassed not only nudity, but also a wide variety of bodily functions, including sex, urination, defecation, and spitting. Peter Stallybrass and Allon White argue that the Victorian bourgeoisie, in an effort to convince themselves and others that they belonged to "a different, distinctive and superior class," embraced Descartes' mind-body dualism as a metaphor for social relations. To be respectable, in other words, was to be governed by reason rather than by biology. Members of the middle class, they suggest, believed that bodies and bodily functions should be hidden from public view and that poor people were incapable of disciplining and properly covering their own bodies.[30]

While some believed that parks and gardens could help to civilize the poor, others feared that those who were insufficiently refined to appreciate nature would defile it by their presence. Although access to parks expanded with time, the upper classes long received special privileges. Regent's Park, St. James's Park, and Kensington Gardens, all ostensibly open to the public, barred entry to people who were not "well-behaved and properly dressed."[31] In 1889 one working-class newspaper argued that as Regent's Park was "public property," all classes, not just "fashionable promenaders," should be allowed free access to it.[32] Another way that the wealthy monopolized space—which prefigured Robert Moses' twentieth-century parkways in New York that were designed with bridges too low to allow the passage of buses on which poor people, particularly poor black people, rode—were restrictions that conferred exclusive access to many of "the most agreeable drives of London" to privately owned carriages.[33]

Isabella Gladstone condemned these restrictions, arguing that public parks and gardens "must really be open, open to all, the shabbiest denizen of the crowded street as well as the most respectable occupant of the suburban villa."[34] In sharp contrast to her perspective, some maintained that the parks of London required even greater restrictions than already existed. In an 1887 letter to the *Standard,* the author of a book on vagrancy demanded that "the practice of men and women lying together on the grass should be absolutely prohibited." He went on to assert that "filthy and verminous" individuals should be ejected from parks and forcibly "disinfected."[35] The newspaper took up the issue in earnest, asserting the next day that the parks were being taken over by "hulking ruffians and disorderly women," who spent their days "sleeping, swearing, fighting, and occasionally indulging in other practices which are a scandal and an offence. The result is that all decent people are driven from their vicinity, and practically debarred from the use of the Parks as long as they choose to infest them . . . even when they are gone they leave their traces behind them, and reduce the fresh sward to such a condition that it becomes unfit to be walked upon or sat upon, or to be played upon by children."[36]

The London County Council, an elected body that succeeded the Metropolitan Board of Works in 1889, quickly assumed responsibility for many of the parks and playgrounds in the metropolis. In the process, it promulgated a series of regulations that were intended not only to enforce respectable behavior, but also to prevent places intended for recreation from being sullied by productive uses. The first person to chair the council's parks and open spaces committee was none other than Reginald Brabazon (known from 1887 as the twelfth Earl of Meath). Under his direction, the council prohibited "drying clothes, beating carpets, washing clothes and dogs, sorting rags . . . committing acts of indecency or nuisances of any kind, distributing or selling articles, collecting money for other than a public object, misusing water-closets or urinals, playing games except where allowed, playing musical instruments, fishing without authority, holding public meetings except on the sites set apart for the same . . . [and] practising gymnastics without proper authority." In 1893, seeking to extend its control to the shaping of musical taste, the London County Council hired a "musical adviser," to whom the programs of all park band concerts were to be submitted for prior approval.[37] Even if all of these regulations were enforced uniformly on all classes of visitor—a highly unlikely supposition—the burden they imposed fell most heavily on working-class individuals, who often possessed no other places in which to carry out the proscribed activities.

PATHOLOGY

Concerns about the body, urban green space, and empire came together in late nineteenth-century London around fears of degeneration: the theory that individual human beings, or successive generations, could become more primitive as time passed. As Meath put it, if nothing were done to ameliorate the unhealthy conditions of urban life, they might "ultimately lead to a degeneration of the race and to national effacement." Because boys growing up in the slums of "darkest London" were the soldiers and sailors of the future, Meath believed that unhealthy urban conditions threatened to undermine Britain's imperial power. To him, playgrounds and playing fields were vital elements in ensuring that Britain remained the most powerful country in the world.[38]

Most commentators believed that degeneration primarily affected poor and working-class individuals. Those who asserted that the lower levels of society were degenerating disagreed about what caused it and why it afflicted poor people more than wealthy ones. Some observers suggested that people of different social classes were biologically distinct and that poor people carried a "hereditary predisposition to break down under the depressing effects of town life." Others blamed the phenomenon on the unhealthy environment of cities, in which large numbers of individuals spent their lives in "the vitiated atmosphere of confined workshops" and in narrow, poorly ventilated streets.[39] Regardless of whether they understood degeneration to be caused by heredity or environment, its adherents shared a conviction that members of the working class were physically and morally inferior to their social superiors.[40]

The miasmatic theory of disease, which dominated discussions of public health until the 1880s, played an important role in shaping the environmental interpretation of degeneration. It posited that illness was induced by breathing air that was contaminated with the products of decaying vegetable or animal matter, such as garbage, sewage, and dead bodies. Each year, miasma was blamed for killing thousands of Londoners by unleashing a deadly process of decay within their bodies. Far greater numbers, though spared illness and death, were thought to suffer irreparable harm nonetheless. In the words of one medical authority, air that was contaminated by putrefaction "must inevitably deteriorate or destroy the general health and bodily vigour."[41]

Many middle- and upper-class Victorians assumed that insalubrious urban environments degraded not only the bodies but also the morals and behavior of poor and working-class people. This assumption was embraced by the sanitary reformer and M.P. Lyon Playfair. In an address to the Social Science Congress in 1874, he argued that "crowded and unhealthy" environments led inexorably to "low morals and low intelligence." In such places, he declared, "The condition of human beings is scarcely above that of animals—where appetite and instinct occupy the place of the higher feelings."[42] Five years later one of the leading members of the Kyrle Society made a similar assertion, declaring that "an intimate connexion" existed "between crime and unhealthy conditions of living."[43]

According to some, the only cure was to leave the city, either temporarily or permanently. This might involve moving to the suburbs, charitable programs that sent children from the slums on summer holidays in the countryside, or even emigration to uncrowded continents across the seas. Others argued that instead of fleeing the city, people should work to increase the amount of accessible green space within it. To prevent "race deterioration," argued the physician John Edward Morgan, cities had to be made healthy by improving their air. "Cellar dwellings should be closed up, courts and alleys cleared out, and the sites which they occupied left open to serve the double purpose of air-shafts and play-grounds."[44] Although many argued that public parks, gardens, and playgrounds would purify poor and working-class people both biologically and morally, others disagreed, maintaining that government had no business interfering in the real estate market and that poor people, rather than benefiting from exposure to green space, would contaminate it by their presence and diminish its enjoyment by those who could truly appreciate it: the middle and upper classes.

Fears of degeneration reached a crescendo during the second Anglo-Boer War (1899–1902), when many commentators attributed Britain's military difficulties to the allegedly poor health and slight stature of its soldiers. Such allegations, whipped up in large part by Lord Meath, generated enormous political pressure on the government to do something. It responded in 1903 by appointing the Inter-Departmental Committee on Physical Deterioration. Testifying before the committee, the social investigator and reformer Charles Booth claimed that poor health among the "lower classes" could be traced primarily to "bad sanitary conditions, insufficient fresh air, and insufficient opportunity of getting out of town into the country."[45] The committee's report shared Booth's assessment. Rejecting the claims of eugenicists that the urban working class was genetically inferior to the rest of society, the committee recommended that greater attention be given "to the preservation of open spaces with an abundance of light and air."[46]

CONCLUSION

Visitors to London are often impressed by the amount of green space that it contains. Those with an awareness of the high cost of land in the metropolis may marvel that so much valuable real estate was saved for the public good. Viewed from this perspective, the existence of parks, playgrounds, and gardens within one of the world's largest and most densely populated cities might be construed as the triumph of beneficence or governmental compulsion over the values of the marketplace. Yet the process by which many green spaces in London came to be preserved was far more complex. Although it often included a struggle between those who owned land and those who did not, it just as frequently pitted landowners against one another.

Far from opposing the creation of additional parks and gardens, many property owners supported the idea enthusiastically—as long as it did not cost them anything. Few were willing to sell their land at a price below the market rate, but everyone recognized that its value would increase sharply if their neighbors' land became protected from development. Efforts to save green space also provided a way for both upper-class commoners and aristocrats to portray themselves as supporters of the downtrodden. In 1884 one newspaper speculated that the recent interest that several members of the House of Lords had shown in open spaces was little more than a cynical attempt to "pose as champions of the classes who have recently been agitated to demand the abolition of the Second Chamber."[47] Many advocates of green space no doubt shared Octavia Hill's belief that the safeguarding and opening of common land would "give a share in his country to be inherited by the poorest citizen," and that it would unite in "joyful fellowship" people of "different natures, different histories, and different anticipations."[48] This belief that green space would help to engender social stability echoed the earlier efforts of Edwin Chadwick to promote sewerage systems rather than economic redistribution as the proper response to poverty.[49] For others, including the Earl of Meath and many members of the Metropolitan Public Gardens Association, the creation of playgrounds in Britain's crowded capital was crucial to ensure that its inhabitants were fit—both morally and physically—to fulfill their responsibilities as an imperial people.

In contrast to today, when many environmentalists—at least in the United States—idealize "wilderness" as the purest form of nature, Victorians viewed this term with far greater ambivalence. For many, the ideal landscape was not a wilderness, but a garden. This understanding owed much to the Bible, particularly its account of the Garden of Eden and God's injunction to Adam and Eve to exert dominion over creation. Such cultivation and control, summed up by the Victorian concept of improvement, was frequently applied not only to the environment, but also to human behavior. In this view, wild places and wild conduct were both associated with humanity's expulsion from the original garden. Parks and playgrounds were designed to expose the inhabitants of crowded cities to nature in a form that was both physically and morally salubrious, but if proper care were not taken, the experience might result in injury, disease, or moral contagion. Similar attitudes pertained to the human body, which seemed to teeter precariously on the divide between nature and culture.[50]

At first glance, the playground that the Metropolitan Public Gardens Association opened in the spring of 1884 might seem to have had little in common with the prison that preceded it. Considered more closely, however, important similarities emerge. Both institutions were carefully bounded places in which people in positions of power deployed elaborate regulations and surveillance to discipline the bodies and the minds of the people within them, with the goal of preventing disorder and strengthening society.

Notes

Research for this project was supported in part by a Junior Faculty Research Grant from the University of North Carolina at Charlotte and by a Faculty Grant from the Southern Regional Education Board. I am grateful to the editor and to all who offered feedback when I presented earlier versions of this essay at the Shelby Cullom Davis Center for Historical Studies at Princeton University, 12–13 December 2003, and at the Third Round-Table on Urban Environmental History at the University of Sienna, 24–27 June 2004.

1. *Times* (London), 6 May 1884, p. 9f; *Pictorial News*, 8 May 1884; *Illustrated London News*, 10 May 1884. This playground later became known as the Newington Recreation Ground.

2. *Times* (London), 11 September 1884, p. 8a. During its first couple of years the group was called the Metropolitan Public Garden, Boulevard, and Playground Association, but for the sake of consistency this essay uses the name that it adopted shortly after it transformed the Horsemonger Lane Gaol into a playground in 1884. On the work of this group and its allies, see S. Martin Gaskell, "Gardens for the Working Class: Victorian Practical Pleasure," *Victorian Studies* 23 (Summer 1980): 479–501; Howard LeRoy Malchow, "Public Gardens and Social Action in Late Victorian London," ibid., 29 (Autumn 1985): 97–124; Hazel Conway, *People's Parks: The Design and Development of Victorian Parks in Britain* (Cambridge: Cambridge University Press, 1991), esp. pp. 212–14.

3. B. R. Mitchell, *British Historical Statistics* (Cambridge: Cambridge University Press, 1988), p. 25.

4. Octavia Hill, "More Air for London," *Nineteenth Century* 23 (February 1888): 181–88, esp. p. 182.

5. Isabella M. Holmes (née Gladstone), "Green and Grey London," *Sunday Magazine,* 1888, p. 268.

6. Asa Briggs, *Victorian Cities* (1963; reprint ed., Berkeley: University of California Press, 1993), pp. 314–17; Jonathan Schneer, *London 1900: The Imperial Metropolis* (New Haven, Conn.: Yale University Press, 2001), esp. pp. 17–36.

7. Ouida, "The Streets of London," *Woman's World* 1 (1887–88): 481. On its fascinating author, see Terry Coleman, "Outrageous Ouida," in *The Victorians: A World Built to Last,* ed. George C. Perry and Nicholas Mason (New York: Viking, 1974), pp. 226–27.

8. Ouida, "Streets of London," p. 484.

9. Henry W. Lawrence, "The Greening of the Squares of London: Transformation of Urban Landscapes and Ideals," *Annals of the Association of American Geographers* 83 (1993): 90–118, esp. p. 114. Despite all of the changes that have occurred in London during the past dozen decades, some of its squares still remain inaccessible to the public.

10. *Evening News and Post,* 4 September 1890.

11. *Daily Telegraph,* 13 March 1885.

12. *Daily News* (London), 12 April 1884, p. 7.

13. *Reynolds's Newspaper,* 13 May 1888, p. 3.

14. *Daily Chronicle,* 26 July 1888.

15. London County Council, *London Parks and Open Spaces* (London: London County Council, 1924), pp. 50–51.

16. *Daily News* (London), 17 April 1884, p. 6.

17. Alicia M. Cecil, *London Parks and Gardens* (New York: Dutton, 1907), p. 218.

18. David Owen, *The Government of Victorian London, 1855–1889: The Metropolitan Board of Works, the Vestries, and the City Corporation* (Cambridge: Harvard University Press, Belknap Press, 1982), pp. 147, 150.

19. "Garden Party at Parliament Hill, Hampstead," *Graphic,* 8 August 1885, 143; *City Press* (London), 30 March 1889, supp., p. 1.

20. "Hampstead Heath Extension," *Graphic,* 30 March 1889, p. 318.

21. Cecil, *London Parks and Gardens,* p. 194.

22. On the early history of the Kyrle Society, see the *Times* (London), 6 April 1931, p. 6.

23. Octavia Hill, "Space for the People," *MacMillan's Magazine* 32 (August 1875): 329.

24. *Times* (London), 10 July 1883, p. 8f.

25. *Daily Chronicle,* 13 October 1884.

26. "Playgrounds for Children," *Queen,* 30 September 1884.

27. *Echo,* 30 July 1885.

28. Blanche Medhurst, "Playgrounds and Open Spaces," *Woman's World* 1 (1888): 511.

29. *Times* (London), 14 November 1849, p. 4e.

30. Peter Stallybrass and Allon White, *The Politics and Poetics of Transgression* (Ithaca, N.Y.: Cornell University Press, 1986), p. 202.

31. *Report of the Select Committee on Public Walks* (1833), p. 5, quoted in Lawrence, "Greening of the Squares of London," p. 111.

32. *Reynolds's Newspaper,* 28 April 1889, p. 3.

33. *Truth,* 28 March 1889, p. 571. On Moses' parkways, see Robert A. Caro, *The Power Broker: Robert Moses and the Fall of New York* (New York: Knopf, 1974), pp. 318–19, 951–54.

34. Isabella M. Gladstone, "The Public Garden," *Eastward-Ho!* 4 (March 1886): 442.

35. *Standard* (London), 5 September 1887, p. 2.

36. Ibid., 6 September 1887, p. 5. For an interesting examination of this attitude, see Nan H. Dreher, "The Virtuous and the Verminous: Turn-of-the-Century Moral Panics in London's Public Parks," *Albion* 29 (Summer 1997): 246–67.

37. London County Council, *London Parks and Open Spaces,* pp. 73, 76. On Meath's activities, see F. H. A. Aalen, "Lord Meath, City Improvement, and Social Imperialism," *Planning Perspectives* 4 (1989): 127–52.

38. Reginald Brabazon, "Decay of Bodily Strength in Towns," *Nineteenth Century* 21 (May 1887): 674.

39. John Edward Morgan, *The Danger of Deterioration of Race from the Too Rapid Increase of Great Cities* (London: Longmans, Green, and Co., 1866), p. 11.

40. Robert Jones, "Physical and Mental Degeneration," *Journal of the Society of Arts* 52 (1904): 337; Daniel Pick, *Faces of Degeneration: A European Disorder, c. 1848–c. 1918* (Cambridge: Cambridge University Press, 1989), esp. p. 218; Gerry Kearns, "Biology, Class, and the Urban Penalty," in *Urbanising Britain: Essays on Class and Community in the Nineteenth Century,* ed. Gerry Kearns and W. J. Withers (Cambridge: Cambridge University Press, 1991), pp. 12–30; Kelly Hurley, *The Gothic Body: Sexuality, Materialism, and Degeneration at the Fin de Siècle* (Cambridge: Cambridge University Press, 1996).

41. George Alfred Walker, *Gatherings from Graveyards* (London: Longman, 1839), pp. 239–40.

42. Lyon Playfair, "Pure Air, Pure Water, and Pure Soil," *Builder* 32 (10 October 1874): 846.

43. *Times* (London), 8 October 1897, p. 11f. For an interesting discussion of this belief, see Chris Otter, "Making Liberalism Durable: Vision and Civility in the Late Victorian City," *Social History* 27 (Jan. 2002): 1–15, esp. p. 2.

44. Morgan, *Danger of Deterioration,* p. 50.

45. Inter-Departmental Committee on Physical Deterioration, *Minutes of Evidence,* Cd. 2210 (1904), ¶1075; Bentley B. Gilbert, "Health and Politics: The British Physical Deterioration Report of 1904," *Bulletin of the History of Medicine* 39, no. 2 (1965): 143–53; Richard A. Soloway, *Demography and Degeneration: Eugenics and the Declining Birthrate in Twentieth-Century Britain* (Chapel Hill: University of North Carolina Press, 1990), pp. 44–47.

46. Inter-Departmental Committee on Physical Deterioration, *Report,* Cd. 2175 (1904), pp. 85–86.

47. *Metropolitan,* 29 November 1884.

48. Octavia Hill, "The Future of Our Commons," *Fortnightly Review* 28 (November 1877): 641.

49. See Christopher Hamlin, *Public Health and Social Justice in the Age of Chadwick: Britain, 1800–1854* (Cambridge: Cambridge University Press, 1998).

50. Bruce Haley, *The Healthy Body and Victorian Culture* (Cambridge: Harvard University Press, 1978), esp. p. 70.

3

The War on Rats versus the Right to Keep Chickens

Plague and the Paving of San Francisco, 1907–1908

Joanna L. Dyl

The disease must be built out of existence. This is the hope of San Francisco and in time that city will be one block of concrete throughout, and the gateway to the Orient closed against plague.

—Dr. Rupert Blue, U.S. Marine Hospital Service, 1908

In the aftermath of the April 1906 earthquake and fire, rubble filled the streets of San Francisco's burned district. The disaster had destroyed 28,000 buildings, initially rendering 200,000 people homeless. Many found residence outside the burned district, while others settled in cheap, flimsy wooden structures that sprang up to fill the demand for everything from housing to warehouse space. They were among the lucky ones as tens of thousands of San Franciscans remained in refugee camps and tent cities in parks and other open spaces through the fall and winter. Sanitation often took a back seat to survival as citizens struggled to restore a semblance of civilized life. In the days after the disaster, the bodies of more than five hundred dead animals, mostly horses and cows felled by collapsing buildings, lay strewn about the city. Garbage went uncollected, and with the city's incinerator damaged, the rapidly accumulating waste had to be shipped out to sea, with seven hundred loads departing daily. Water remained in short supply for months, and sewer pipes lay in pieces.[1] Some of the residents of the city found the new conditions to their liking, however—San Francisco's rat population, never small, thrived in the chaos of the post-disaster city.

In 1907, the situation went from bad to worse when health officials discovered bubonic plague in the city. Driven by fears of economic marginalization, San Francisco's commercial and political elites mobilized the citizenry to combat plague. Ultimately, they fought the plague on ecological grounds, and the campaign that became known as the "war on rats" concentrated on making the city inhospitable as rat habitat. The modern material of concrete replaced wood over millions of square feet of both private and public property. Strict sanitary regulations enforced a distance between the city's human residents and the animals and plants that provided their food. As Augustin Keane declared in a 1908 account of the fight against the plague, San Franciscans believed that antiplague measures and reconstruction after the earthquake and fire would make San Francisco the "first twentieth-century city" and "probably the world's most sanitary city."[2] The actions of San Francisco's city officials and business leaders in 1907 and 1908 reflected an attempt to implement their vision of the modern city through infrastructural and sanitary improvements. Although many of these changes benefited all San Francisco residents, the city's poor and recent immigrants suffered disproportionate burdens in undertaking modernization efforts.

THE FIRST OUTBREAK, 1900–1904

The 1907 outbreak was not the first appearance of bubonic plague in San Francisco. On 6 March 1900, a forty-one-year-old Chinese lumber salesman named Wong Chut King died in the basement of the Globe Hotel in the heart of Chinatown. An autopsy and subsequent bacteriological tests revealed that he had died of plague. Over the next four years, the disease struck 121 people in San Francisco, 90 percent of them Asian. This racial breakdown made it easy for San Franciscans to continue their long tradition of using the Chinese as scapegoats in times of medical or economic crisis.[3] The appearance of the bubonic plague was no ordinary health crisis, however. The disease had resulted in millions of deaths in China and India since its reappearance on the global stage in the 1860s, augmenting its reputation as one of history's deadliest killers. Quarantines of ports affected by the disease had disrupted international trade as well as local economies. Ultimately, the discovery of plague in San Francisco in 1900 led localities from New Orleans to Sydney, Australia, to refuse to admit either products or passengers coming from California.[4]

In 1900, many San Franciscans hoped that if they denied the plague's existence, it would simply disappear. Two out of the city's three daily newspapers refused to acknowledge the disease. Politicians also sided with the forces of denial, and medical authorities were divided on the question. San Francisco's status as the economic hub of the Pacific coast was the centerpiece of its image, and city leaders already worried about declines in manufacturing and the growth of Pacific rivals such as Los Angeles and Seattle. A plague-induced quarantine threatened to severely disrupt San Francisco's trade-based economy. Working people also doubted that rumors of bubonic plague were true, preferring to believe those who claimed that the disease had not touched their city. Even many Chinese, subjected to both drastic antiplague measures and suspicious deaths, doubted the diagnoses of white medical authorities. Their familiarity with the devastation wrought by plague in China made them question claims that this mild outbreak represented the same disease—and provided added incentive to deny that plague afflicted their community. Even the inevitable quarantine of San Francisco's port appeared to be of only minor concern to the working people of the city. In the weekly *Coast Seamen's Journal,* the newspaper of the powerful Coast Seamen's Union published in San Francisco, the quarantine of California in 1900—like most quarantines of ports—rated only a one-sentence mention.[5] Not until February 1903 did all parties involved officially concede that plague existed in San Francisco.

Even while the plague's presence remained disputed, San Francisco's health authorities acted to contain the epidemic. Health officer Joseph Kinyoun first attempted to physically confine the plague to Chinatown by quarantine, but a judge ruled the barrier to be illegal and racially discriminatory. City officials then employed fumigation and disinfection to cleanse the Chinese district. Laborers flushed Chinatown's sewers and filled them with sulfur gas. They cleared garbage from streets and alleys and deposited chloride of lime in its place. Floors and walls were scrubbed and sprayed with a solution of bichloride of mercury, and as the State Board of Health explained, "all the dark rooms, alleyways, and stairways were subjected to a coat of whitewash." Symbolically and in terms of sanitation, health officials were whitening the darkness of Chinatown. Disinfecting activities were limited to the seventeen blocks recognized as Chinatown, with reports emphasizing that it was never necessary to "invade" the adjacent white neighborhood.[6] However, these efforts failed to halt either plague cases or deaths.

On 6 February 1904, the City and State Boards of Health, the San Francisco Board of Supervisors, and the Marine Hospital Service jointly passed a resolution that called for the ratproofing of Chinatown. The resolution required the destruction of "all cellars, basements, and underground places." Those that were to be rebuilt had to be rebuilt with concrete. Improvements affected a total of 625 parcels of real estate in Chinatown (only sixteen of which were owned by Chinese). Looking back from the vantage point of 1909, contemporary historian Frank Morton Todd concluded that these efforts had successfully "built out" the plague from San Francisco and only the special circumstances following the earthquake and fire allowed the disease to return.[7] Todd's knowledge of the 1907–8 campaign colored his perspective on the earlier outbreak, but the 1900–1904 efforts nevertheless made drastic changes in the physical structure of Chinatown.

During this first outbreak, medical authorities were only guessing at the epidemiology of the plague. Some suspected that rats were connected to the disease, but the uncertainty meant that efforts to combat the plague were based on guesses, rather than knowledge, as to how it spread. W. H. Kellogg reminisced that in 1900, "we knew the rat was important, but we did not proceed as if we did."[8] Only in 1905 did experiments by the Indian Plague Commission demonstrate that fleas transmitted the bubonic plague between rodents. When rats died of the plague, their fleas would seek out another host, and humans contracted the plague when bitten by infected fleas.[9] When the 1907 outbreak barely touched Chinatown, it forced many San Franciscans to accept, or at least consider, this new scientific alternative to their earlier racialized explanations of the disease.

In fact, the reason for the plague's relatively light death toll in San Francisco in comparison to Asia probably had little to do with either sanitary conditions in the city or measures taken to combat the disease. When a flea bites an infected animal (or human) it ingests the plague bacilli along with the blood that it feeds upon. Inside the flea, enzymes from the plague organism form a blood clot blocking the flea's stomach. This clot allows plague germs to grow but also blocks new meals from reaching the flea's stomach, causing it to bite more aggressively in an attempt to dislodge the ball of blood. Each bite injects plague into the skin of the flea's victim. If the flea cannot dislodge the clot of blood, it will starve, becoming another victim of the plague. Different species of flea are more susceptible to these plague-induced clots. The Asian rat flea, *Xenopsylla cheopis,* is particularly vulnerable, but *X. cheopis* was less common in San Francisco than *Nosoophyllus fasciatus,* the northern European rat flea, which transmits the plague only one-third as efficiently as *X. cheopis.* This quirk of ecological luck is the most likely explanation for why San Francisco's bubonic plague epidemic claimed only hundreds rather than thousands of victims.[10]

THE RETURN OF THE PLAGUE

Despite San Francisco's previous experience with plague, the return of the disease caught the city unprepared. On 27 May 1907, a seaman named Oscar Tomei died of plague in U.S. Marine Hospital Service custody. He had lived on board a tug in the bay for the previous five or six weeks, coming ashore to eat at a lodging house near the waterfront. At first, Tomei's seemed like an isolated case, but on 9 August, Ida Costi and her husband Francesco, an Italian couple who lived in a crowded building on Telegraph Hill, were diagnosed with the disease, and three days later, plague took the life of the Russian sailor Alex Rubrek. By the end of the month, health authorities had identified fourteen human cases and found infected and dead rats at various sites along the waterfront and around the city. The epidemic would only worsen over the next few months, ultimately killing 89 people out of 167 total cases.[11] The plague peaked in September, October, and November 1907, before the cold, rainy weather sent rats deeper into hiding and reduced the number of fleas to spread the disease.

The first attempts to make sense of the return of the dreaded disease relied on the old associations of disease with Chinatown. These assumptions about plague quickly encountered the reality that it was white people, not Chinese, who were dying in 1907. Even though Chinatown had burned in the 1906 fire, cement foundations constructed during the 1904 outbreak survived. An expert observer, Richard H. Creel, described Chinatown as "by far the most sanitary district in the city of San Francisco from a structural point of view," and Chinatown's near immunity provided evidence of the efficacy of fighting the disease by altering the built environment. Ultimately, the 1907 plague epidemic affected every district in the city except the outlying Sunset and Richmond districts, where the population density was relatively low.[12]

Evidence indicates that the plague struck San Francisco's poorer citizens and recent immigrants most heavily. The Board of Health Report for 1907–8 described the nativity of seventy-two of the victims. Sixty-one percent were foreign-born, almost twice the percentage in the city's population as a whole. The primary foci of the disease, including the Latin Quarter, Lobos Square, and areas along the waterfront, were home to poor white San Franciscans.[13] Starting in September, eighteen cases struck the Lobos Square refugee camp, which housed two thousand people, a high percentage of them Italian, in newly constructed two-room wooden cottages. These "earthquake cottages" lacked running water and shared communal bathing facilities; they also had no foundations to keep rats from gaining access. The shortage of housing in San Francisco after the earthquake and fire meant that exorbitant rents forced poor people to scramble for shelter, making it more likely that they would find themselves living in close proximity to rats. For example, many of San Francisco's Italian residents who escaped the refugee camps lived in hastily thrown-together shacks that Creel described as "ideal rat harbors." The crowded Latin Quarter, home to mostly working-class Italian immigrants, was the site of as many as half the total plague cases. Among the working class and poor, recent immigrants—with Italians being the largest group—were thus most susceptible to both the disease and efforts to reconstruct the urban environment to counter it.[14]

The official interpretation of the plague de-emphasized questions of social class and ethnicity in favor of scientific sanitation and structural change—"building out" the plague. Stories of plague cases focused on contact with rats rather than on race or class. Deaths among the Bowers family of the Mission District were traced to a funeral the family's two young sons had held for a dead rat found in a cellar. A doctor and his family became infected after opening a wall to investigate a "foul odor" and finding rat cadavers.[15] Todd's official account of the campaign declared that most of the victims were respectable white people, "subsisting on a generous diet and dwelling in houses that would commonly be called 'sanitary,'" and referred to the plague as a "danger that was common to all parts of the City." Keane explicitly attributed the infection of the Lobos Square refugee camp to its proximity to a stable rather than to inherently unsanitary living conditions among the refugees.[16] Blaming rats and the urban environment, rather than any group of people, served to universalize the danger and engage more San Franciscans in the campaign against the plague.

This seemingly scientific perspective inspired a citywide "war on rats" that demanded the participation of and sacrifices from all citizens. Observers like Creel and William Colby Rucker of the U.S. Marine Hospital Service recognized that totally eradicating the rat from San Francisco would prove impossible because survivors would reproduce more quickly.[17] The key to victory for humans was to eliminate sources of food and rat habitat—what today we might refer to as changing the ecology of the city. Rats had thrived for hundreds of years in urban environments, but the new ideals of sanitation and the new technologies of concrete held out hope that a war against rats could lead the rodents to be "built out of existence" in early twentieth-century San Francisco.[18] In practice, poor people, particularly those of marginalized ethnicities, bore the brunt of the combat between San Francisco's people and its rats. Surveillance by health inspectors, criticism of practices such as the keeping of chickens, and the expenses of meeting new structural requirements all fell most heavily on San Francisco's working-class residents.

MOBILIZING AND PAVING THE CITY

In 1907, unlike in the earlier outbreak, neither city nor state officials attempted to deny the existence of plague in San Francisco. Mayor Edward R. Taylor, himself a trained physician, requested federal assistance, and the U.S. Marine Hospital Service sent Dr. Rupert Blue, architect of the 1904 cleanup of Chinatown, to oversee the fight against the disease. One of the first crises facing the campaign was finding a place to house the sick. During the month of August, cases were brought to the City and County Hospital, which the Board of Health bitterly described as "an old, dilapidated, most unsanitary wooden structure, erected as a temporary hospital thirty-five years ago and used ever since in spite of repeated condemnation by successive Boards of Health." On 12 and 13 August, the hospital treated four plague patients, and an elderly Irish orderly named Jeremiah O'Leary contracted the disease from one of them. In late August, two more hospital employees took sick, and on the twenty-seventh, a patient who had no signs of plague upon admittance developed the disease.[19] The hospital was infested with both rats and plague. Doctors constructed a "rat-proof galvanized iron fence sunk in concrete" around the infectious disease pavilion; they did the work themselves when laborers "threw down their tools and refused to come near the building."[20] Ultimately, the hospital had to be demolished and burned. The fate of San

Francisco's public hospital demonstrated that the city's practice of modern sanitation and provision of medical care remained very much a work in progress. The 1907 outbreak of bubonic plague galvanized changes—like the construction of a new hospital—more broadly needed for urban public health.

City leaders mobilizing the community to constructive action against the plague did not have an easy task. The chief surgeon of the Isolation Hospital, Arthur O'Neill, observed in his report that "the very name 'plague' seems to strike terror into the hearts of the community," and the panic shown at the infestation of the hospital was not an isolated instance.[21] At the same time, throughout the fall, health officials encountered what William Hobdy, a colleague of Blue's with the U.S. Marine Hospital Service, described as "the apathy of the public and the studied indifference of the press" when asked to take specific measures against the disease. For the medical experts heading the plague campaign, panic seemed a more appropriate reaction than apathy. In December 1907, 1.4 percent of rats inspected for plague were infected, a percentage as high as in the worst epidemics of modern times.[22]

Faced with a brief winter in which to address the problem of infected rats or face an even greater outbreak in the spring, Dr. Blue and the Board of Health called a meeting of leading citizens in early January. San Francisco's business and political elites did not perceive the same crisis that the medical community did. Blue sent out six hundred invitations, but only sixty men attended the meeting. However, those who did adopted a resolution calling on Mayor Taylor to appoint a Citizens' Health Committee to mobilize the populace. The committee consisted of twenty-five members, twelve with medical degrees. Once these community leaders and experts were on board, the campaign for a widespread "war on rats" began to gain momentum. The committee collected more than $177,000 from corporations and individuals, with which it employed four hundred inspectors and laborers, purchased countless rat traps and vast quantities of poison, paid bounties to rat catchers, and printed 700,000 circulars and pieces of literature.[23] At least one observer considered Dr. Blue's efforts to involve the entire community to be crucial to the success of the campaign; Augustin Keane praised Blue for not using his individual authority to quarantine the city but instead for his efforts to "bring the citizens of San Francisco into the ranks of his workers."[24]

As in the 1900 plague outbreak, the primary concern of San Francisco's merchants and businessmen was the potential economic impact of the plague. Observers in San Francisco and elsewhere in the Bay Area believed that they had learned a lesson from the earlier epidemic—the existence of plague in a city need not "of itself seriously threaten" commerce as long as the community took "prompt and vigorous action" against the disease.[25] The Citizens' Health Committee organized ten committees and forty-two subcommittees representing various industries and social and fraternal organizations, each charged with communicating the urgency of antiplague efforts to its constituency.[26] The subcommittees adopted aggressive scare tactics centered on the threat of quarantine. A card posted in drugstores throughout the city threatened that "though you may have business to attend to now, you certainly will have none to bother you should the City be quarantined." Almost 300,000 copies of a circular declaring that quarantine "would be a death blow to the industrial life of the city" were distributed in three languages.[27] The health risks posed by the plague—when they were mentioned at all—took a backseat to the economic threat.

In the spring of 1908, San Francisco was "a city of meetings"—a total of 162 meetings over six weeks to educate and mobilize the population. Schoolchildren heard presentations and took home "kitchen cards" with measures for getting rid of rats. A questionnaire given to ten thousand employees of large businesses included the question, "Have you succeeded in convincing your neighbors that San Francisco is facing a real danger, not only of a sanitary nature, but more particularly of a vital commercial and financial nature?" This question illustrates not only the attempt to involve the entire citizenry in the campaign of education and surveillance, but also the judgment that the financial threat from plague was greater than the sanitary one.[28] Ministers preached rat destruction and cleanliness in their churches, and saloon keepers posted notices in their establishments. Butchers and produce dealers were warned that housewives would not patronize any "butcher shop, vegetable stall or fruit stand that was not clean and wholesome."[29] The committee published circulars in Italian and Greek as well as English to reach San Francisco's immigrant populations, many of whom lived in relatively insular, non-English-speaking communities. Literature was also translated into Japanese for publication in Japanese-language newspapers. San Francisco's various labor organizations fully backed the campaign, with the San Francisco Labor Council, the Building Trades Union, and the City Front Federation all forming subcommittees. Walter Macarthur, the editor of the *Coast Seamen's Journal,* was even a member of the executive committee.[30] By involving labor, circulating literature widely, and publishing in several languages, the campaign set out to enlist all San Francisco's residents—men, women, and children alike—in the war on rats.

The effect of the massive campaign to mobilize the citizenry of San Francisco was to exacerbate the problem that plague posed for working-class residents of the city. Initially the disease represented another in a long list of threats to their health that menaced individuals, their families, and friends and neighbors every day. Fewer San Franciscans died of the plague in 1907–8 than of tuberculosis, typhoid fever, or diphtheria.[31] However, the "war on rats" expanded public health demands placed on San Franciscans. Suddenly, inspectors invaded their homes and businesses, insisting that they change daily practices and pave their property. These demands most dramatically affected recent immigrants, particularly Italians, many of whom came from rural backgrounds and gravitated to employment in familiar fields such as fishing, farming, selling produce at the market, and driving horse-drawn scavenger wagons. These residues of rural life—industries seen as insufficiently urban and modern—became the targets of the campaign to sanitize San Francisco into a modern city.[32] At times, individuals benefited when landlords and the city installed plumbing and sewers for their use. In other cases, they watched as their homes were torn down in the name of sanitation and their employment saddled with new restrictions.

Doctor Blue's "war on rats" consisted of five components: trapping, poisoning, exposing to natural enemies, cutting off food supply, and eliminating habitat. Blue and his assistants divided the city into thirteen sanitary districts, each headed by a surgeon with a small army of inspectors, assistant inspectors, foremen, and laborers at his disposal. At its peak, the effort employed 919 men and trapped 13,000 rats in a single week.[33] Bounties of five cents per rat, later increased to ten cents, encouraged trapping. Bounties also helped ensure that the extent of disease among the city's rodent population could be monitored since the bodies were brought to the campaign's headquarters and inspected for the presence of plague. A new law required city residents to place traps and allowed for a fine of five hundred dollars per day or six months in jail for violations. Over 200,000 rats died in traps, and thousands more were poisoned. Many of these animals "died in the sewers and were washed into the bay, where they could be seen floating in rafts near the outfalls."[34] Thousands of rat corpses floating in San Francisco Bay hardly seems characteristic of a successful sanitary campaign, but reducing the existing rat population was only part of Blue's strategy.

In theory, the combination of changing human practices and altering the physical environment of the city would transform San Francisco from ideal to inhospitable rat habitat. One report explicitly referred to the need to "render rodent life as difficult as possible."[35] In order to encourage these changes, the Board of Supervisors passed a series of ordinances addressing unsanitary practices and structures. Floors in basements had to be made of concrete, and foundations had to be built of concrete, brick, or stone and extend at least one foot above the ground. Obviously, both older frame houses and new wooden dwellings thrown up after the fire rarely met these requirements. In total, health officials destroyed 1,713 houses and disinfected 11,342. The houses condemned and torn down were almost exclusively the homes of the poor, many of whom had lost their previous residences in the fire and now lost those they had scrambled to reconstruct in the wake of the disaster. In total, 6,433,100 square feet of the city of San Francisco—including basements, stables, chicken yards, and sidewalks—were rebuilt with concrete.[36]

Citywide, inspections resulted in 82,554 abatement of nuisances notices. Yellow placards marked premises that failed to meet the new standards, and newspapers published convictions for sanitary offenses. These methods of shaming persuaded most people to improve their property—only 370 arrests took place—but some resisted the unexpected and often prohibitive expense. In Butchertown, the owners of hog pens initially refused access to rat catchers. Todd stated that there were hundreds of cases in which "it was extremely difficult to convince the owner that his innocent plank wall or bit of flooring was a danger."[37] Some property owners reverted to claims that plague did not exist in the city when given notice that a rat harbor existed on their property; perhaps some citizens genuinely believed that the disease was merely an excuse for authorities to impose hardships on them.[38] Others marshaled different arguments. Members of the Builders' Exchange initially greeted the Citizens' Health Committee demands with the statement that rats "follow civilization and cannot be driven away."[39]

The vast mobilization campaign played a role in pressuring San Francisco residents to cooperate with the sanitation campaign, as did the evidence that the Board of Health possessed the political and legal authority to condemn their property. The forces of the "war on rats" sometimes dealt with resistance to cleanup efforts by simply barging into the premises in question and beginning the work. Perhaps most importantly, the courts initially supported the Board of Health's claim of broad powers to abate rat harbors as sanitary nuisances.[40] The Citizens' Health Committee, with its ties to virtually every industrial organization in the city, also served as a "mediator between the authorities and the citizens who were required to spend considerable sums of money" to make their homes and businesses conform to new sanitary regulations.[41] Evidence indicates that the vast majority of the paving undertaken by the "war on rats" took place on private property, and it was therefore most likely paid for by private funds. Of the more than six million square feet of concrete laid, sidewalks made up less than 5 percent while basements and other floors consisted of 67 percent, stables 18 percent, and chicken yards 11 percent.[42] Private citizens in San Francisco spent an estimated one million dollars to ratproof their property. Supporters of the campaign believed that this "immense outlay of both money and labor" was essential, however, to achieve their goal of permanently eradicating plague from the city.[43]

Separating the Urban and the Rural

The modernization of San Francisco to make it a more sanitary city consisted of several components. Paving the city with concrete was one. Another involved choices about the place of animals in the urban environment. Obviously rats were to be excluded from the modern city. Cats and dogs, on the other hand, were allowed as useful companions. Horses remained essential work animals, but the new antiplague ordinances established a distance between horses and humans that had not existed before. Wooden houses constructed with stables as the ground floor were condemned as a plague hazard. Todd described "the ordinary stable" as a "complete rats' boarding house," and he and Keane both blamed several plague cases on stables in close proximity to human dwellings. When San Francisco instituted formal regulations governing ratproofing in stables, the city had 5,292 stables. The Stable and Carriage Owners' Association formed an active subcommittee of the Citizens' Health Committee and persuaded stable owners to install 3,967 concrete floors. Another 903 stables were temporarily ratproofed on the condition that they be torn down within two years. Over 400 stables were eliminated entirely from the city, sometimes along with the houses built over them.[44] The earthquake and fire represented a turning point in the replacement of horses with automobiles in San Francisco, and the ratproofing of stables and the paving of the city contributed to that process.

While horses remained as work animals, food animals were almost entirely exiled from the city in the wake of the plague. The Board of Health found "chicken coops and other places where live animals were kept" to be "dangerous harboring and breeding places for rats," and chicken coops became the target of a special ordinance.[45] San Francisco was home to some sixteen thousand domestic chicken yards, mostly located in thinly settled suburbs and in the densely populated poorer quarters of the city, where Todd described them as "thick among the houses." Chickens were an important element in the subsistence strategy of poor families. In 1904, a dozen eggs cost an average of 23 cents, ranging from 19 to 45 cents depending on the season, and eggs were staple ingredients in most meals. Chickens could also provide a source of meat, and a successful backyard chicken farmer could earn extra income by selling eggs and young chickens to neighbors. Chickens were kept in yards and fed grain and table scraps, which sanitary officials suspected supported as many rats as fowl.[46] The 1908 ratproofing ordinance required that chicken yards have a concrete floor and be surrounded by a brick or concrete wall at least a foot high and by a six-foot wire net. Such elaborate chicken coops were prohibitively expensive for most practitioners of the domestic chicken industry, and eleven thousand people were forced to dispose of their birds. Those with the financial resources to remain in the business covered their chicken yards with a total of 676,000 square feet of concrete and gravel.[47]

San Francisco's working poor resisted the loss of their chickens. Frank Morton Todd facetiously observed that "sacred among the palladia of American liberty is [the] right to keep chickens." As a proponent of the sanitary measures, Todd was mocking the vehemence with which people defended their right to raise chickens on their property. He went on to list the factors that made chicken yards "one of the most troublesome problems" facing the ratproofing campaign. Specifically, Todd referred to "the number, the varying intelligence, and the temperamental diversities of the people that keep chickens—their passive resistance, and infinite stratagems, and degrees of 'pull' when threatened with prosecution." His defamation of the character of people with chickens in their yards demonstrated the class conflict that lay beneath the surface of a plague campaign in which sanitation officers inspected and judged the homes of working-class people, many of them immigrants.[48] Some were successful in their resistance, and the Board of Health's campaign to rid San Francisco of chickens did not end with the "war on rats." Four years later, in 1912, the board reported that 275 chicken yards containing 3,213 chickens had been shut down after a round of inspections while another 69 had been remodeled.[49]

The closing down of San Francisco's domestic chicken yards went hand in hand with the rise of industrialized chicken factories in the greater Bay Area, particularly Petaluma. As early as 1894, Petaluma's exhibit at the Midwinter Fair in San Francisco featured the new technology of incubators. The Petaluma Incubator Company—"'progression' is our motto"—sold incubators, brooders, and other chicken farm equipment nationwide. Petaluma boosters believed that the chicken industry would make their city "the leading manufacturing city of the Pacific Coast," surpassing even San Francisco, and half a million hens already lived there in 1895. In 1912, the California Chicken Company opened in Mayfield, just thirty-two miles south of San Francisco, with ambitions to put "the chicken raising business on a business basis." They emphasized the "remarkable cleanliness" of their operation, which resulted from "the underlying principles of sanitation rightly applied."[50] Exiling chickens from San Francisco thus opened up the urban market to these large companies located in nearby rural areas. It was also part of a broader and ongoing process in which food production became disconnected from the city.

The dairy industry was another food industry gradually driven from the city. As recently as 1902, San Francisco's chief sanitary inspector worried that suburban growth meant that dairies and cattle raising were moving outside the bounds of the city and county, where they were no longer subject to inspection. Most dairies were owned by Italian and Swiss immigrants who had only short-term leases on their land, and the demand for land in the aftermath of the fire led to a 50 percent reduction in the number of dairies in San Francisco between June 1907 and June 1909. The city no longer worried about dairies leaving the city; in fact, a 1910 ordinance regulated the keeping of cattle "with a view to clearing out all of the dairies within the city limits." Because of the Bay Area's moderate climate, milk was rarely iced in transit, and approximately 130 dairies remained within one hundred miles of the city, most located across the water in more rural Marin County. Nevertheless, San Francisco had taken another step in gradually distancing itself from its food supply.[51] This time the process was driven less by fear of the plague than by the geographical expansion of the urban area, exacerbated by the earthquake and fire.

San Francisco's stables not only housed horses and cattle but also contributed to a cycle in which the city's excess manure fertilized rural gardens in southern San Francisco County and adjacent San Mateo County that provided the urban center with vegetables and fruit. As in many of the industries targeted in the "war on rats," Italian immigrants made up a high percentage of both these farmers and the men who transported vegetables and manure to and from the city.[52] The plague brought scrutiny to this practice of "truck and garden farming," which appeared to be unsanitary. Dead rats were discarded with stable manure, and then, as Todd described it, "the vegetable grower's wagon stops at the barn on its way back from market, [and] loads up on manure and bubonic rats" before returning to the farm. In response to the threat of the spread of plague, the State Board of Health prohibited the transport of manure from San Francisco to other counties. Truck farmers faced with losing a significant portion of their income countered with a threat "to shut off . . . the City's supply of green vegetables." Stable owners were left with no easy means of disposing of manure and added their objections to the new law. Ultimately, a compromise allowed manure to be sent out only in metal-lined wagons "from stables certified to be sanitary and equipped with rat-proof manure bins." The cost of inspection would be born by the San Francisco Gardeners' and Ranchers' Association.[53] In this case, the sanitary regulations, rather than protecting the city, focused on preventing the spread of plague from the city to the vulnerable countryside. The effect of these restrictions on the cycle of city manure fertilizing rural gardens was to further separate the urban and the rural, the city and the farms that provided sustenance to its population.

The paving of San Francisco during the "war on rats" involved laying a total of almost 6.5 million square feet of concrete, including sidewalks, basements, floors, stables, and chicken yards, but constructing a rat-proof city was a long-term process.[54] In fiscal year 1911–12, the Board of Health reported that 1,308 houses and 406 stables were destroyed as antirat measures, the same year that an additional 275 chicken yards were shut down. Even between 1918 and 1920, "animals removed from premises" remained a significant sanitary violation, with over one hundred cases each year.[55] San Francisco's poor continued to be subjected to the loss of their homes and livelihoods in the name of sanitation even as they simultaneously benefited, at least in part, from a more healthful urban environment.

SANITIZING THE CITY

Post-disaster San Francisco faced a challenge in disposing of refuse produced by its human residents as well as its animal ones. Under a privatized system of garbage collection, licensed scavenger wagons, mostly owned and manned by Italian immigrants, made individual arrangements with householders along their routes. The high rates they charged provided an incentive for residents to find illicit means of disposing of their waste. Scavengers in turn had to pay to have their collections incinerated at the Sanitary Reduction Works, the company with an exclusive franchise to dispose of the city's refuse, so some found unofficial means of dumping their cargo. As early as 1903, the Department of Public Health described the city's system of garbage collection as "neither scientific nor sanitary" and suggested municipal garbage collection as the solution. The situation became even worse after the fire, with scavengers often surreptitiously depositing garbage on the suddenly abundant vacant lots.[56] When human garbage collectors failed to complete their jobs, rats stepped in as natural scavengers. The first step in eliminating garbage as a food source for the city's rats was to reform residents' methods of disposing of their waste. Women led the campaign to educate the community about the importance of using metal garbage cans with lids that sealed tightly. As part of the "war on rats," the city distributed fifty thousand new garbage cans.[57] The new regulations and strict enforcement of garbage collection most affected people for whom scavenging represented a subsistence strategy. Licensed professional scavengers were one such group, but another would have been the poorest of the poor, who utilized the waste prevalent in any urban environment. Thus, the crackdown on garbage—like that on chicken coops—closed some of the loopholes exploited by the city's poor in their struggle to eke out a living.

Although in San Francisco the plague outbreak provoked the city to strictly regulate garbage disposal, San Francisco's experience paralleled a nationwide trend in which professional sanitary engineers began to take over municipal refuse programs in the early twentieth century. They persuaded public health officials that technology could solve garbage disposal problems.[58] In San Francisco, the technological panacea was the construction of a new municipal incinerator. Citizens passed a bond initiative in May 1908 that allocated one million dollars for the project. Despite promises that the new incinerator would not spew noxious odors, not surprisingly none of the city's residents wanted it in their neighborhood. The pollution from the existing plant spread over a half-mile radius, and the earthquake and fire had forced more people to move to the vicinity, leading to a noticeable increase in the number of complaints. Two new sites were eventually selected, and by June 1913, an incinerator in the Islais Creek District, in the Outer Mission, finally neared completion. (Ironically, this neighborhood on the southern outskirts of the city was home to many of the vegetable gardens that supplied produce to San Francisco.) However, the plant operated only intermittently as the city sought reimbursement from the contractor for failing to meet guarantees that it wouldn't emit odors, gases, smoke, or dust.[59] The technological solution to the problem of solid waste disposal had fallen short.

Damage to San Francisco's sewer system presented another major sanitary crisis in the wake of the 1906 disaster. In fact, the system had been in crisis for virtually its entire existence. San Francisco's sewers had expanded steadily from 128 miles of mains in 1880 to 307 in 1900, but this increase represented expansion to incorporate growing suburbs as much as improvements in coverage of the central city.[60] Perhaps the worst location was Channel Creek, the former Mission Creek—widely referred to as "shit creek"—which ran through the lumberyards, warehouses, and factories of the Mission District. Captain Fred Klebingat described the creek as "an open sewer . . . as thick as soup." The rumor among the longshoremen was "if you took two gulps of that stuff it would be the end of you." The Citizens' Health Committee reported that nearby lumberyards and warehouses swarmed with rats.[61] In 1900, the Board of Public Works developed a systematic plan for sewers and drainage in the city, and a bond issue to provide funding passed in 1903. The process of construction had barely begun, however, when the earthquake shattered many of the main sewage pipes and dislodged the line and grade of others. The authorities in the "war on rats" considered the sewers to be the "great highway" of rats as well as a source of "protection, food, and drink" for them. Broken sewers provided rats with easy access to an underground network running throughout the city and connecting wealthy areas with poor ones.[62]

In 1908, over 125 sewer outlets discharged their contents along the bay shore. Waste backed up in blocked outlets and behind bulkheads, and none of the sewers were screened to prevent rats from entering. At Polk and North Point Streets near Fort Mason, sewage flowed out for 250 feet over the ground. The Citizens' Health Committee concluded that the existing sewer system was "a terrible menace to public health" and supported a bond issue that allocated another four million dollars for improvements to the system.[63] The new system reduced the number of outlets discharging along the shoreline to four and located those remaining points at places where powerful tidal currents would sweep the waste out to sea. The stated goal was "no perceptible pollution of the waters of the bay." In the aftermath of the earthquake, fire, and plague, San Francisco's campaign against rats joined with a growing concern with water sanitation to provide the impetus for improvements to the city's sewer system.[64]

Removal of sewage outfalls was not the only improvement the waterfront needed to meet San Francisco's new standards for sanitation. As one of the few areas to survive the fire, the waterfront remained in its original makeshift state. Most wharves were constructed of wood and offered no protection against rats. Because the plague spread via ships, the waterfront represented a particularly important site in the "war on rats." The Citizens' Health Committee feared that, unless waterfront conditions improved, all the resources expended in the "war on rats" would be wasted as the disease would easily reenter the city. They proposed "the installation of a concrete seawall, bulkheads, and properly constructed modern piers" along with the improvements to the sewer system.[65] These planned structural improvements were accompanied by practices intended to prevent rats from traveling between ships and shore, including installation of funnel-shaped metal rat guards on the lines anchoring ships to docks, regular disinfection and fumigation of ships to kill rats on board, and inspection of cargo.[66]

The focus on the waterfront and vessels that constantly passed through San Francisco's port not only protected the city but also sought to avoid infecting the countryside. William Hobdy described his work overseeing the fumigation of all kinds of vessels, from trans-Pacific liners to lumber trawlers to passenger ferries and steamboats, as a constant effort to "prevent the spread of the Plague from San Francisco to the various Bay and river ports that are now so intimately connected." San Francisco's place at the center of regional trade networks meant that rat-borne urban disease threatened the entire Pacific coast. Shipowners and captains were as sporadically cooperative as other groups affected by the campaign. Hobdy frequently reported ships escaping from the harbor without undergoing disinfection, particularly when their destination ports were too small to have harbor authorities to check if vessels had been certified rat-free. He also complained of insufficient staff to patrol the waterfront and enforce measures to stop rats from traveling between ships and shore.[67]

THE PERSISTENCE OF PLAGUE

The initial efforts of Hobdy and others to contain the plague were futile, as San Francisco was not the only Bay Area city stricken with plague in 1907–8. Across the bay in Oakland the percentage of infected rats was as high as in San Francisco, although there were only twenty human cases. In fact, while the plague lay dormant in San Francisco between 1904 and 1907, the only cases in the region were three in Contra Costa County and one in East Oakland.[68] The source of infection in rural areas of the East Bay was contact with ground squirrels, which had presumably been infected with the disease by rats from shipyards. In 1908, researchers confirmed that ground squirrels in Contra Costa were dying en masse from the plague, the first confirmed epizootic among wild animals in North America. The widespread infection among ground squirrels—seventeen hundred infected squirrels were found in the years after 1908—threatened any hopes of containing and eradicating the plague. However, once Blue and his associates believed that they had the disease under control in San Francisco, they launched an ambitious campaign to create a "10-mile squirrel free zone" around population centers and to eradicate the disease among ground squirrels across the bay.[69]

Not surprisingly, this campaign would prove as unsuccessful as Hobdy's earlier attempts at containment. Plague remained consistently ahead of its pursuers, spreading from county to county even as the squirrel body count exceeded 700,000. By 1912, infected squirrels were found in nine California counties. Plague-positive squirrels repeatedly turned up in counties believed to be free of the disease.[70] The campaign to eradicate plague among California's rodents did have an interesting sidelight. One U.S. Department of Agriculture biologist, David E. Lantz, suggested that rodent populations were so large because humans "killing off the natural enemies of rodents" had "disturb[ed] natural conditions." Lantz advocated an end to bounties on predators such as hawks, owls, foxes, and coyotes. He even suggested that hawks and owls should have "legal protection" because of their value as rodent predators.[71] There is no evidence that Lantz's suggestions were acted upon, but they indicate that the plague sparked early ecological thinking in the attempt to make the city and the countryside alike inhospitable to rodents.

The plague did not return to San Francisco after 1908, but it periodically resurfaced in other California cities. One case developed in Los Angeles that year, and thirteen cases were scattered among six northern California counties between 1910 and 1914. An outbreak of pneumonic plague, the more virulent form of the disease, struck Oakland in 1919 and killed thirteen out of fourteen victims. The first patient had been squirrel hunting in the foothills of Alameda County just before coming down with the disease. In another example of an unprepared medical community, the disease was not diagnosed as plague until after six people had died.[72] In 1924–25, pneumonic plague broke out among a Mexican community in Los Angeles and claimed more than forty lives. In an echo of San Francisco's treatment of Chinatown, four low-income Mexican neighborhoods were quarantined and twenty-five hundred homes damaged or destroyed in the effort to contain the disease. Overall, including the San Francisco epidemics, California suffered a total of 372 plague cases and 257 deaths over the period from 1900 to 1925.[73]

Although individual cities could be made less susceptible to plague, the disease established a permanent foothold in western North America. Plague-infected squirrels have been found in fifteen western states. Wild rodents, particularly ground squirrels, became a reservoir from which the disease has occasionally spread to other species of animals or infected humans. Such reservoirs, which also exist in Asia and Africa, are believed to be the source of the pandemics that have earned plague its reputation as a global killer. Isolated cases continue to occur in the United States. Small epidemics occurred in 1975–76, 1980, and 1983, with the 1983 epidemic involving forty cases. Most of the victims contracted the disease in rural New Mexico and many of them were Navajo.[74] Despite the best efforts of health authorities in the early years of the twentieth century to contain the disease, plague escaped their control and became a permanent part of the ecology of the United States.

In 1907, the bubonic plague frightened San Francisco politicians and business leaders who saw it as an economic threat, as well as health officers who perceived the disease to be a new danger to lives in the city and the nation. The public health crisis of the plague outbreak provided an opportunity to mobilize a broad base of citizens behind a particular vision of the city's future, one dominated by concrete and commerce. The alliance of community elites and health authorities made the plague a problem for the entire population of the city, human and animal, through the "war on rats." House-by-house inspections and ordinances covering everything from chicken coops to basements intruded on the lives of working-class people.

Although accounts of the "war on rats" couched the campaign in neutral terms of sanitation and targeting of rodents, the process of constructing a modern, sanitary city had differential impacts on San Francisco's population because of class and ethnic differences in living conditions. Sanitizing the city meant changing how people lived, altering not only the built environment but also the daily practices of urban residents to approach new idealized expectations for the twentieth-century city. Recent immigrants, particularly San Francisco's large Italian population, were most likely to be employed in industries affected by the new measures as well as to live under conditions that made them targets for sanitary improvements. Working-class residents and members of marginalized ethnic groups benefited from improved sanitation, but thousands lost their homes as well as elements of their subsistence strategies, such as chickens in the backyard.

The "war on rats" transformed the ecology of San Francisco, not only for rodents but for humans as well. The campaign may have fallen short of Dr. Blue's goal of transforming the city into "one block of concrete throughout," but it did accelerate the modernization of San Francisco in the form of a new sewer system, improved garbage collection, and the replacement of wooden structures with "rat-proof" concrete ones. Part of this transformation was the increasing exclusion of animals and other rural elements from the urban environment as the modern city compartmentalized the natural and the urban. For example, the "war on rats" shut down the domestic chicken industry and interrupted the use of manure from San Francisco to fertilize the suburban farms that produced food for the city. As a result, the city became increasingly isolated from food production in the name of sanitation. Although environmentalists may look back with nostalgia on a city more integrated with its hinterland, those changes did make San Francisco a healthier place for all its human residents.

NOTES

Epigraph: Rupert Blue, "The Underlying Principles of Anti-Plague Measures," reprinted in *Eradicating Plague from San Francisco: Report of the Citizens' Health Committee and An Account of Its Work,* ed. Frank Morton Todd (San Francisco: Press of C.A. Murdock & Co., March 31, 1909), p. 218.

1. Report of the Board of Health, *San Francisco Municipal Reports for the Fiscal Year 1906–07* (San Francisco: Neal Publishing Co., 1908), pp. 515–16. All reports by the Board of Health and Board of Public Works are from the *Municipal Reports* for a given year unless otherwise stated. The exact names of the agencies vary (i.e. the Department of Public Health is renamed the Board of Health) and report titles therefore vary slightly as well.

2. Augustin C. Keane, "San Francisco's Plague War," *American Review of Reviews* 38, no. 5 (November 1908): 561.

3. Racial data are available for 92 out of 121 cases, primarily those from 1900 to 1902. Of the victims for whom information is available, 87.0 percent were Chinese. The addition of five Japanese women who contracted the disease (four of them prostitutes in the same house) shows that 92.4 percent of victims were Asian. This contrasts sharply with the 1907 epidemic. For recent histories of disease in San Francisco's Chinatown, including the plague outbreaks, see Susan Craddock, *City of Plagues: Disease, Poverty, and Deviance in San Francisco* (Minneapolis: University of Minnesota Press, 2000); and Nayan Shah, *Contagious Divides: Epidemics and Race in San Francisco's Chinatown* (Berkeley: University of California Press, 2001). For a journalistic but insightful account of the plague in San Francisco, see Marilyn Chase, *The Barbary Plague: The Black Death in Victorian San Francisco* (New York: Random House, 2003). Earlier discussions include: Silvio J. Onesti, Jr., "Plague, Press, and Politics," *Stanford Medical Bulletin* 13, no. 1 (February 1955): 1–10; Guenter B. Risse, "'A Long Pull, A Strong Pull, and All Together': San Francisco and Bubonic Plague, 1907–1908," *Bulletin of the History of Medicine* 66 (1992): 260–86; Joan B. Trauner, "The Chinese as Medical Scapegoats in San Francisco, 1870–1905," *California History* (Spring 1978): 70–87.

4. Vernon B. Link, *A History of Plague in the United States of America,* Public Health Monograph No. 26 (Washington, D.C.: U.S. Government Printing Office, 1955), pp. 1–2; Mike Davis, *Ecology of Fear: Los Angeles and the Imagination of Disaster* (New York: Vintage Books, 1998), pp. 251–52. Craddock, *City of Plagues,* p. 132.

5. On reactions among the press and medical journals, see Onesti, "Plague, Press, and Politics," pp. 2–4. On the reaction among the Chinese, see Shah, *Contagious Divides,* pp. 134–48. *Coast Seamen's Journal* 13, no. 38 (1900): 4.

6. Report of the State Board of Health, "The Disinfecting, Cleaning, and Fumigating of Chinatown, in the City and County of San Francisco, State of California" (27 August 1901), pp. 37–40.

7. Resolution quoted in Trauner, "The Chinese as Medical Scapegoats," p. 80. Todd, *Eradicating Plague,* p. 32.

8. W. H. Kellogg, "Rodent Plague in California," *Journal of the American Medical Association,* 14 September 1935, p. 856.

9. Rupert Blue, "Rodents in Relation to the Transmission of Bubonic Plague," in *The Rat and Its Relation to the Public Health* (Washington, D.C.: Government Printing Office, 1910), p. 146. This describes the transmission of the most common form of the plague, the bubonic form. The more deadly pneumonic variation can spread from human to human via bacilli located in the sputum.

10. Chase, *The Barbary Plague,* pp. 190–91. Charles T. Gregg, *Plague: An Ancient Disease in the Twentieth Century,* rev. ed. (Albuquerque: University of New Mexico Press, 1985), pp. 76–78. One study found 68 percent of fleas in San Francisco were

N. fasciatus and only 21 percent were *X. cheopis* (three other species made up the remainder). Link, *A History of Plague,* pp. 20–21.

11. Walter M. Dickie, "Plague in California 1900–1925," pamphlet reprinted from the proceedings of the Conference of State and Provincial Health Authorities of North America, 1926, pp. 30–32; Todd, *Eradicating Plague,* pp. 38–40; Chase, *The Barbary Plague,* p. 151; Risse, " 'A Long Pull, a Strong Pull, and All Together,'" p. 268; letters of William C. Hobdy, May and August 1907, vol. 32, Record Group 90, Public Health Service, National Archives and Records Administration, San Bruno, Calif; Link, *A History of Plague,* p. 20. The exact number of cases and deaths attributed to the plague varies slightly in different reports.

12. Craddock, *City of Plagues,* pp. 149–50; Rupert Blue, "The Campaign Against Plague in San Francisco, California," in Todd, *Eradicating Plague,* pp. 291–93; Richard H. Creel, "Rat Proofing as an Antiplague Measure," in *The Rat and Its Relation to the Public Health,* p. 172 (quote). Only eight of the victims in the 1907–8 outbreak were Chinese. Trauner, "The Chinese as Medical Scapegoats," pp. 80–81.

13. Board of Health Report, 1907–8, pp. 632–33. Ninety percent of the victims in this sample were described as white.

14. Creel, "Rat Proofing as an Antiplague Measure," p. 172. On the large Italian population at Lobos Square, see Hanna Astrup Larson, "Enrichment of the Refugees," *San Francisco Call,* magazine section, 20 October 1907.

15. Blue, "Rodents in Relation to the Transmission of Bubonic Plague," p. 259; Chase, *The Barbary Plague,* pp. 164–66.

16. Todd, *Eradicating Plague,* pp. 9, 141; Keane, "San Francisco's Plague War," pp. 568–69.

17. William Colby Rucker, "Rodent Extermination," in *The Rat and Its Relation to the Public Health;* Creel, "Rat Proofing as an Antiplague Measure," p. 173.

18. Blue, "The Underlying Principles of Anti-Plague Measures," p. 218.

19. Board of Health Report, 1907–8, pp. 481–88; Chase, *The Barbary Plague,* pp. 152–53.

20. Ibid., pp. 481, 486, 588.

21. Ibid., p. 588.

22. Letter from William C. Hobdy to Surgeon General, 28 February 1908, vol. 34, Record Group 90, Public Health Service, National Archives and Records Administration, San Bruno, Calif.; Gregg, *Plague: An Ancient Disease,* p. 87.

23. Todd, *Eradicating Plague,* pp. 7–10, 42–51, 86–88. The committee ultimately did not need all of its funds and returned a dividend of 19 percent to all subscribers. Todd described "the saving of the City from quarantine" and the dividend as the main accomplishments of the committee (ibid., p. 154). Chase, *The Barbary Plague,* pp. 170–72.

24. Keane, "San Francisco's Plague War," p. 571.

25. *Report of the Committee of the Society of Sigma Xi on the Plague Conditions in Berkeley, San Francisco, and Oakland* (Stockton, Calif., March 1908), pp. 6–7. This document reported on plague conditions and responses to the disease in cities throughout the Bay Area. It urged that Berkeley follow the lead of San Francisco and act aggressively to prevent the plague from taking root there.

26. Todd, *Eradicating Plague,* pp. 59–70.

27. Documents reprinted ibid., pp. 211, 199.

28. Ibid., pp. 81, 121, 207; Link, *A History of Plague,* pp. 14–15.

29. Todd, *Eradicating Plague,* pp. 72–75 (quote p. 75), 110–17.

30. Ibid., pp. 91–101, 104–7, 161; *Labor Clarion,* 14 February 1908. It is worth noting that 270,000 circulars were published in English and only 10,000 each in Italian and Greek (Todd, *Eradicating Plague,* p. 199).

31. Board of Health Report, 1907–8, pp. 598–99. In his book on the 1918 flu pandemic, Alfred W. Crosby writes that "lethal epidemics were not as unexpected and therefore not as impressive in 1918 as they would be today." Crosby, *America's Forgotten Pandemic: The Influenza of 1918* (New York: Cambridge University Press, 1989), p. 319. This would be even more applicable to 1907–8. In the specific case of the plague, the disease's reputation augmented fear in the community, but the fact that relatively few people contracted the disease presumably helped counter that effect.

32. Andrea Sbarboro, "Life of Andrea Sbarboro: Reminiscences of an Italian–American Pioneer" (San Francisco, 1911), p. 192, MSS C-D 1580, The Bancroft Library, University of California, Berkeley; "San Francisco Labor Losses," *Coast Seamen's Journal,* 23 May 1906, p. 2. In his history of public health, John Duffy identifies the need to teach newcomers "how to live in an urban environment," including the necessary sanitary practices, as a theme of U.S. public health history. Duffy, *The Sanitarians: A History of American Public Health* (Urbana: University of Illinois Press, 1990), pp. 2–3.

33. Board of Health Report, 1907–8, pp. 482–83; Todd, *Eradicating Plague,* p. 153. Military rhetoric was omnipresent in accounts of the effort. For example, Keane employed an extended military metaphor in describing the division of the city into districts, each with the hierarchy and discipline of a military unit. Colby Rucker of the U.S. Marine Hospital Service referred to the need to "erect wide systems of municipal fortifications" and described the campaign as "a contest between the wit of man on the one hand and acute animal instinct on the other." Keane, "San Francisco's Plague War," p. 563; Rucker, "Rodent Extermination," pp. 162, 153 (quotes).

34. Rucker, "Rodent Extermination," p. 154; Todd, *Eradicating Plague,* pp. 158–59 (quote), 191.

35. Citizens' Health Committee, *Insanitary Conditions along the San Francisco Water Front: A Report to the Citizens Health Committee of San Francisco by its Water Front Committee,* (San Francisco, 1908), pp. 10–11.

36. Link, *A History of Plague,* p. 18; Todd, *Eradicating Plague,* pp. 141–42, 194.

37. Link, *A History of Plague,* pp. 17–18; Risse, "'A Long Pull, A Strong Pull, and All Together,'" p. 281; Todd, *Eradicating Plague,* p. 141.

38. Todd, *Eradicating Plague,* pp. 165–66. For resistance to cleanup efforts, see Keane, "San Francisco's Plague War," pp. 566–69. Keane mentions the proprietors of hog pens, bakeries, rag dens, and stables as objecting to orders to clean up their premises.

39. Quoted in Risse, " 'A Long Pull, A Strong Pull, and All Together,'" p. 280.

40. Ibid., p. 282. By mid-May 1908, as enthusiasm for the campaign and evidence of infection waned, judges began to dismiss cases against alleged violators of sanitary laws, helping bring the most intense phase of the campaign to a close.

41. Board of Health Report, 1907–8, p. 485.

42. Statistics calculated from numbers in Todd, *Eradicating Plague,* p. 183.

43. Ibid., pp. 165–66; Creel, "Rat Proofing as an Antiplague Measure," pp. 174–75 (quote).

44. Todd, *Eradicating Plague,* pp. 73, 131–34; Keane, "San Francisco's Plague War," pp. 567–69. The quality of stables, like the quality of human housing, had declined in some areas after the fire, with horses being stabled in woodsheds and other small quarters. *San Francisco Daily News,* 27 October 1906.

45. Board of Health Report, 1907–8, p. 485.

46. Todd, *Eradicating Plague,* p. 139 (quote and statistic on number of chicken yards); Creel, "Rat Proofing as an Antiplague Measure," pp. 175–76. For the price of eggs, see California Promotion Committee, *Poultry Raising in California* (San Francisco, 1905). For the prevalence of eggs in contemporary recipes, see *The Refugees' Cook Book* (San Francisco, 1906). For a secondary account, see Craddock, *City of Plagues,* p. 155.

47. Todd, *Eradicating Plague,* p. 140.

48. Ibid., p. 139.

49. Report of Board of Health, 1911–12, p. 621. The fact that not a single one of 344 chicken yards passed inspection indicates that sanitary officials were looking to shut down the city's remaining chicken industry.

50. Petaluma Incubator Co., *Petaluma Incubator* catalog (Petaluma, Calif., 1895), pp. 1–2, 4, 16–17; *The Mammoth Chicken Coop of the Fairmont, St. Francis, and Palace Hotels* (San Francisco, 1912).

51. Report of the Department of Public Health, 1901–2, p. 564; Board of Health Report, 1908–9, pp. 685–86; Report of Board of Health, 1910–11, p. 181; Report of Board of Health, 1911–12, pp. 657–58. On the ethnic composition of the dairy industry, see "San Francisco Labor Losses," *Coast Seamen's Journal,* 23 May 1906, p. 2.

52. Stewart Perry, *San Francisco Scavengers: Dirty Work and the Pride of Ownership* (Berkeley: University of California Press, 1978), p. 16; Joel A. Tarr, "From City to Farm: Urban Wastes and the American Farmer," *Agricultural History* 49 (1975): 605.

53. Todd, *Eradicating Plague,* pp. 131–32 (all quotes); Board of Public Works Report, 1907–8, p. 709.

54. Link, *A History of Plague,* p. 18.

55. Report of Board of Health, 1911–12, pp. 621–24. Department of Public Health, mimeographed list of violations, 1916–20 (San Francisco), folder 10, carton 50, California Department of Industrial Relations, Division of Immigration and Housing Records, BANC MSS C-A 194, The Bancroft Library, University of California, Berkeley.

56. Report of the Department of Public Health, 1902–3, pp. 658 (quote), 664; Board of Health Report, 1907–8, p. 484; Board of Public Works Report, 1907–8, p. 709; Perry, *San Francisco Scavengers,* p. 15. In San Francisco in the early twentieth century, Italians—many of them illiterate—dominated the waste trades. On the prominence of recent immigrants in the waste trades, see Carl Zimring, "Dirty Work: How Hygiene and Xenophobia Marginalized the American Waste Trades, 1870–1930," *Environmental History* 9, no. 1 (January 2004): 80–101. Italian banker and community leader Andrea Sbarboro reminisced that he and other leading Italians in San Franciscans bid for the franchise that became the Sanitary Reduction Works in part to preserve the jobs of their fellow Italian immigrants. Sbarboro, "Life of Andrea Sbarboro," p. 169.

57. Rucker, "Rodent Extermination," p. 160; Todd, *Eradicating Plague,* pp. 110–12, 123–24, 187. Todd estimates 100,000 new garbage cans while Link says it was 49,046 (still "practically one for every home"); Link, *A History of Plague,* p. 18.

58. Martin V. Melosi, *The Sanitary City: Urban Infrastructure in America from Colonial Times to the Present* (Baltimore: Johns Hopkins University Press, 2000), pp. 194–96.

59. Board of Public Works Report, 1907–8, pp. 709–11, 716–19; Board of Public Works Report, 1909–10, p. 546. For evidence regarding nuisance problems with the Sanitary Reduction Works even before the earthquake, see Report of the Department of Public Works, 1904–5, p. 346. Board of Public Works Report, 1912–13, pp. 495–96; Board of Public Works Report, 1913–14, pp. 404–5; Board of Public Works Report, 1914–15, pp. 360–63; Marsden Manson, *Garbage Disposal System. Contract No. 1: For the Construction of Two Incinerating Plants* (San Francisco: Department of Public Works, June 1910). In the long run, San Francisco's community of Italian scavengers successfully resisted a municipal takeover of the industry and formed cooperatives to organize garbage collection in the city. Perry, *San Francisco's Scavengers,* pp. 17–18.

60. Melosi, *The Sanitary City,* p. 153.

61. Quoted in Roger and Nancy L. Olmsted and Allen Pastron, *San Francisco Waterfront: Report on Historical Cultural Resources for the North Shore and Channel Outfalls Consolidation Projects* (San Francisco, December 1977), p. 127. Citizens' Health Committee, "Insanitary Conditions Along the San Francisco Waterfront," 9–10.

62. Link, *A History of Plague,* p. 18; Blue, "The Underlying Principles of Anti-Plague Measures," p. 217 (quote). In *City of Plagues,* Susan Craddock suggests that "the sewer became both the real and symbolic reminder to the upper classes that they could not completely disassociate themselves from the poor and their filth. The sewers transected and thus linked each section of a city whose topographical distinction by this point was a relative degree of class segregation" (pp. 99–100).

63. Citizens' Health Committee, "Insanitary Conditions along the San Francisco Water Front," 8–13 (quote pp. 12–13); Board of Public Works Report, 1913–14, p. 393.

64. Board of Public Works Report, 1913–14, p. 393; Board of Public Works Report, 1907–8, p. 684 (quote). Todd, *Eradicating Plague,* p. 144. Historian Martin Melosi has observed that early underground sewer systems were constructed before the era of germ theory, when discharging sewage into waterways was of little concern. In the late nineteenth and early twentieth centuries, sanitary authorities became concerned with bacteria, although an awareness of the dangers posed by discharge of industrial wastes and toxic materials didn't develop until after World War I. Melosi, *The Sanitary City,* pp. 162–63.

65. Citizens' Health Committee, "Insanitary Conditions along the San Francisco Water Front," 6, 12 (quote); Board of Health Report, 1907–8, p. 486; Rucker, "Rodent Extermination," p. 162.

66. William C. Hobdy, "The Rat in Relation to Shipping," in *The Rat and Its Relation to Public Health,* pp. 209–13; Blue, "The Campaign Against Plague," p. 293.

67. Letters from William C. Hobdy to Surgeon General, esp. 17 September 1907, 2 January 1908 (quote), 28 February 1908, vols. 33 and 34, Record Group 90, Public Health Service, National Archives and Records Administration, San Bruno, Calif.

68. Link, *A History of Plague,* p. 23; *Report of the Committee of the Society of Sigma Xi,* p. 3; Todd, *Eradicating Plague,* p. 231.

69. San Francisco responded to the news of ground squirrel deaths by banning the importation and sale of ground squirrels in the city. Board of Health Report, 1908–9, p. 674; Link, *A History of Plague,* pp. 28–35; Kellogg, "Rodent Plague in California," pp. 1–2; Dickie, "Plague in California," 58 (quote).

70. Kellogg, "Rodent Plague in California," pp. 2–3; Link, *A History of Plague,* pp. 30–35; Gregg, *Plague: An Ancient Disease,* p. 99.

71. David E. Lantz, "Natural Enemies of the Rat," in *The Rat and Its Relation to the Public Health,* pp. 163–69.

72. Dickie, "Plague in California," pp. 32–35; Kellogg, "Rodent Plague in California," pp. 320–21.

73. Dickie, "Plague in California," pp. 39–66; Link, *A History of Plague,* pp. 57–64; Davis, *Ecology of Fear,* pp. 255–58. For a detailed discussion of the Los Angeles outbreak, see William Deverall, "Plague in Los Angeles, 1924: Ethnicity and Typicality," in *Over the Edge: Remapping the American West,* ed. Valerie J. Matsumoto and Blake Allmendinger (Berkeley: University of California Press, 1999), pp. 172–200.

74. Gregg, *Plague: An Ancient Disease,* pp. 5, 233–58.

4

Dead Bodies in Harlem

Environmental History and the Geography of Death

Ellen Stroud

The application to become an official West Harlem "sniffer" betrayed the seriousness of the neighborhood stink. In early 1991, when New York City Office of Environmental Quality Director Michel Gelobter sent a letter to local officials looking for volunteers for the "community-based odor panel," he outlined just how rigorous the selection process would be. In choosing the panel, Gelobter explained, he would have to determine "which individuals have a sense of smell sufficiently sensitive for them to serve on an odor panel," and yet not so sensitive as to be unable to differentiate between mild and noxious fumes.[1]

Potential "sniffers" or "neighborhood noses" would take an odor test, and those who passed would then undergo training sponsored by the city Department of Environmental Protection. Only then would odor panelists be able to complete the official odor log forms properly; otherwise, Gelobter explained, the odor panelists would find it difficult to be confident which box to check when confronted with a long list of twenty-four descriptors that included rotten egg, manure/farmyard, moldy/musty, oily/fatty, putrid/rotting, sewage-like, cabbage-like, raw meaty, burnt rubber–like. The smells of West Harlem were complicated and foul, and to identify and remedy the sources correctly, it would be crucial to distinguish between rotting egg-like smells, rotting meat–like smells, smells of burnt flesh, smells of fresh blood, smells of sewage, of garbage, of mold.[2]

The worst odors in West Harlem came from human bodies. The most pervasive stench came from live bodies: raw sewage from throughout the Borough of Manhattan had been flowing into Harlem since the treatment plant on 145th Street began operation in 1986. By 1991, the city Department of Environmental Quality had acknowledged that design problems were making odor control a serious difficulty at the plant. However, the most disturbing neighborhood smells came from dead bodies. The wealthy, white downtown parish of Trinity Church had opened a crematorium on 153rd Street in the 1970s, and the wretched smell of burning hair and flesh had been sickening Harlem residents ever since. By the 1990s, the neighbors had organized to shut it down, and the sniffing committee would help their cause.[3]

The image of burning bodies was distasteful enough on its own, but the middle- and working-class African American activists painted an even grimmer picture: Trinity Church employees were not just burning corpses in Harlem; they were burning the wrong kind of corpses—the modified bodies of wealthy downtown residents. A modified body is a toxic body, the activists maintained: the odors wafting from the Trinity Church Crematorium were not just the gruesome fumes of burning flesh and bone, but also the toxic vapors of burning mercury from dental fillings, machinery parts from pacemakers, and poisonous gases from the incineration of expensive, varnished coffins.[4]

Though the specifics of their claims were difficult to substantiate, their central insight was true, and surprising: many dead bodies are toxic. The modern dead—and in particular, the modern, wealthy dead—cannot be reduced to mere organic dust and ash; metal joints, surgical materials, mercury dental fillings, silicone breast implants, and pacemaker batteries are all now part of the human machine. Corpse disposal has become newly complex over the course of the nineteenth and twentieth centuries, as human bodies have become more thoroughly incorporated into the industrial world.

Since the mid-nineteenth century, New Yorkers have stubbornly tried to maintain the illusion of a pastoral corpse, but have been repeatedly confronted with its messier nature. Changing bodies, changing ideas about bodies, and new technologies in both the health and the death industries have made it increasingly difficult to hold on to ideas of returning to nature in death. Urban corpses have become part of an industrial landscape, presenting significantly increased risks for death industry workers, offering new hazards for those living near places where bodies are processed and stored, and complicating ways of thinking about the dead. As these changes were taking place in Manhattan, the processing and disposing of bodies was shunted further and further from elite sections of the city, until corpses were all but banished from the island at the end of the twentieth century; the dead body became a waste disposal problem to be sent first to Harlem, and then to the outer boroughs and New Jersey.

The protests against the crematorium in Harlem make these fundamental problems with corpses clear: they are both difficult to dispose of and hard to think about. Dead human bodies should not be industrial pollution, a waste disposal challenge facing the city, another bad smell in a neighborhood plagued by stench. They seem more comfortably pastoral, part of a peaceful and harmonious "nature" in which dust returns to dust. The density of development in Manhattan, however, has made maintaining such illusions impossible. Over the course of the past century and a half, the true "nature" of corpses has repeatedly reminded New Yorkers that dead bodies are messy, dirty, hard to handle, and in relentlessly steady supply.

Participating in the web of nature as food for worms is a disquieting thought, and one that has much to do with the success of the modern funeral industry. Coffins, grave vaults, and mausoleums are designed to keep human bodies separate from even this relatively benign nature for as long as possible. And yet, thinking of dead bodies as hazardous waste is even worse. Corpses, it seems, ought to peacefully return to field and flower; they should not be rotting meat, incinerator ash, or industrial waste. This is the intriguing thing about the crematorium protests: dead bodies were clearly and specifically identified as part of a pollution problem, a particularly gruesome part of the dirt and grit of the city.

New York's corpses are drawing me in many different directions: from the establishment of the earliest churchyard burial grounds, to the development of park-like cemeteries in the mid-nineteenth century, to the changing funeral industry of the early twentieth, to the legal history of body handling and disposal and the peculiar challenges of processing the modern corpse. Each place that I look, I am confronted with both the intellectual puzzle of how New Yorkers have understood what a dead body is and how it should be treated, and also the social and political structures they have put in place to manage the ever-increasing numbers of urban dead.

Paying attention to dead bodies—what they are actually made of, and how they interact with the environments of which they are a part—exposes assumptions about the place of humans in nature, and the place of nature in cities. As dead bodies accumulate in urban places, carefully constructed ideas about control over nature—both within the human body and around it—begin to break down. In this essay, I am beginning an exploration of how people in Manhattan have thought about and disposed of corpses; as I do so, I am arguing that an environmental history of the dead body can lead to new questions and answers about the political, social, and intellectual history of cities.

Death and dead bodies are by no means new subjects for historians, although they are new for those of us who focus on the environment. Historians of medicine, historians of science and technology, and social and political historians have joined sociologists, anthropologists, and others throughout the humanities and social sciences in both historicizing human bodies and crafting a distinguished literature on death.[5] Even a decade ago, sociologist Tony Walter suggested that death had become "the new radical chic."[6] But for all of the focus on the human cadaver and on changes in body disposal and funerary and mourning practices, the human body—dead or alive—has only rarely been considered as a dynamic component of ecological systems.

Environmental historians have recently begun paying much closer attention to the human body, and my work on dead bodies builds on this new scholarship. Most of these new histories have focused on intellectual and cultural themes, investigating how ideas about the nature of bodies have changed over time, and how those ideas have influenced people's interactions with nature. Few have considered the human body as a material, chemical, and biological component of the natural world, with a complex environmental history of its own.

Christopher Sellers was one of the first environmental historians to begin examining the body. In his article "Thoreau's Body: Towards an Embodied Environmental History," Thoreau's body remains almost entirely metaphorical: Sellers asks us to consider how Thoreau's particular social and physical place in the world affected his understanding of and influence on nature. Conevery Bolton Valencius, in her book *Health of the Country,* and Linda Nash, in a recent article in *Environmental History,* continue in this rich metaphorical and intellectual vein, investigating how people's ideas about health, about the functioning of bodies, and about the environmental causes of disease influenced ideas about nature and the shaping of landscapes: settlers drained swamps, planted trees, and irrigated fields to create what they believed would be healthier places for human bodies.[7]

Nancy Langston's research focuses more closely on material histories of bodies, tying physical changes in some fish populations to rising levels of hormones in rivers near cities, which she then links to patterns in the use of synthetic chemicals, possibly including birth control pills. Chemicals enter the human body, are processed, expelled, flushed into the rivers, and then enter the bodies of fish. Human bodies are part of an ecological cycle: there are environmental consequences and environmental histories of eating a hamburger, of washing with soap, of taking medicine. Considering bodies as material components of changing environments, as Langston does, reveals surprising connections between such seemingly disparate developments as the liberating medical advance of the birth control pill and dramatic changes in the bodies of fish, and tells us things we should know—but did not—about our bodies' biological connections to the world around us.[8]

As I follow Harlem's corpses on their complicated and often lengthy path from death to decay, I follow Langston's lead, keeping the focus on the "nature" of human remains, and the complicated interactions between that very messy nature and the urban past. Corpses and their disposal have shaped the environments of which they are a part, and have environmental histories of their own.

I begin with the crematorium protests because they bring the challenges of thinking about corpses as components of the urban environment into high relief: despite what Harlem residents understood as a clear, visible, odoriferous problem, they initially had difficulty convincing officials that there was anything wrong. When residents complained that body processing at the Trinity Church Crematorium was polluting their neighborhood, the operators of the crematory insisted that the odors were imaginary, and that the idea of bodies polluting the air was absurd. When bodies are cremated, crematory supervisor Al Spagnoli explained, they are not so much burned as they are vaporized by extreme heat. According to Spagnoli and other experts, cremated bodies are burned at temperatures exceeding fourteen hundred degrees Fahrenheit, and the resulting emissions from crematory chimneys are nothing but water vapor. And this crematorium was a modern facility, they maintained, complete with air scrubbers to make absolutely certain no foul particles or smells polluted the neighborhood. "It's all psychological," insisted Spagnoli. But neighbors believed otherwise.[9]

"We are going to picket," said Shirley Clarke, who lived near the crematorium. "We want to hold up the hearses, and have signs saying 'We can smell your mother burning.'" The demonstrations staged by neighborhood activists turned out to be more respectful in the end, but nevertheless drew both crowds and attention. "Join the Protest Mass March and Rally Against the Big Stink," read the flyers plastered around the neighborhood in September of 1991 under the sponsorship of four churches, two state senators, two city council members, two U.S. congressmen, and many community organizations. "Demonstrate against poison and odors spewing from North River Sewage Treatment Plant, Trinity Church Crematorium, and Penn Station's MTA Amtrak West Side Trains." One protester used her video camera to capture the black plume coming out of the crematory smokestack, the odor panel did its work, and dozens of neighborhood activists pressured the city to stop the smells. By October, not much had changed at the Amtrak station or the sewage treatment plant, but the crematorium had been closed for good.[10]

The campaign to close the crematorium was successful for three reasons. First, unlike the Amtrak station and the sewage treatment plant, the target was relatively small: a cremation facility burning an average of four bodies a day. Second, there was an identifiable problem at the crematorium: inspectors found that the furnaces frequently malfunctioned, often failing to reach the fourteen hundred degrees Fahrenheit required to burn bodies without fumes. The necessary repairs to remediate the problem were prohibitively expensive, and Trinity Church chose instead to close the facility down. Third, and most interestingly, the rhetoric the activists used to draw attention to the problem was strangely compelling.[11]

An official with the New York State Department of Environmental Conservation initially dismissed the neighbors' complaints, saying "It's not more hazardous to the health any more than if you were right next to a barbecue," a flip characterization that offered no comfort to residents. "It smelled like someone was grilling a barbecue," agreed crematory neighbor Jeanette Perry. "Grilling flesh."[12] But recent scientific studies, court decisions, and legislative initiatives have given credence to the broader claim: that the bodies were not merely dust turning to dust, but rather complicated amalgams of flesh, embalming fluid, and machine turning to toxic ash.[13]

As unpleasant as they are, sewage and transportation exhaust have become accepted, expected hazards of city living. Such hazards are not equitably distributed, frequently placing a heavier burden on poor or minority neighborhoods than on neighborhoods where residents wield more power and privilege. One reason that the city has been slow to respond to Harlem residents' complaints about the Amtrak trains and the sewage treatment plant has been the general understanding that such grittiness is part of urban life. But New Yorkers have not been ready to add body disposal to the inevitable industrial hazards of city living. A corpse should not be just pollution.[14]

It has been a long struggle in Manhattan to keep the dead from polluting the city, one that has meant seeking new ways to mask the biology of the corpse. Early Manhattan residents worked hard to maintain the illusion that their dead were peacefully and gracefully returning to the earth. Early churchyard burial grounds were places of contemplation and repose, small retreats from the growing cacophony of urban development. Very quickly, though, biology broke the illusion. There were simply too many bodies. In 1823, the city forbade the creation of new burial grounds in lower Manhattan, and there were few spaces remaining in those already established. As the churchyards filled, and as fears of concentrations of rotting bodies as sources of miasmas and disease grew during the cholera epidemics of the mid-nineteenth century, urban reformers were pushing to get dead bodies away from the city center.[15]

Trinity Church had been established in 1697 at the tip of Manhattan, and was surrounded by one of the oldest burial grounds in the borough. By the 1830s, the pressure on the churchyard was intense. By 1838, it was impossible to be buried in the Trinity Churchyard unless you had not only been a member of the congregation, but also had a parent, brother, sister, husband, wife, or child already buried there. Church administrators began searching for a new place of burial, and were intrigued by the possibilities of the new "rural" cemeteries, the precursors to our modern landscaped parks.[16]

Mount Auburn Cemetery, established in Cambridge in 1831, and Laurel Hill, in Philadelphia in 1836, were among those cemeteries consciously designed as pastoral landscapes that would offer city dwellers places for "country" walks and picnics, and spaces for contemplating the orderliness of nature. At the same time, and more importantly for Trinity at this juncture, they offered burial space for dead bodies away from the congestion of downtown, a place where bodies could again be part of a peaceful landscape. In a rural cemetery, New York corpses would no longer be sources of disease and controversy, but would rather be back in their "proper" place, in balance with nature.[17]

By 1842, Trinity Church administrators found an appropriate site in upper Manhattan: a parcel of twenty-three acres along the Hudson River, between 153rd and 155th Streets. They purchased the land at once, and set in motion plans to build a fence, a chapel, and a keeper's lodge, and directed the cemetery committee that the land should be "planted with care."[18]

The cemetery was planned as a pastoral place, a rural retreat. It was in a part of the city that was not yet urban, where the wealthy had estates, and which offered privileged urban dwellers the chance to escape and enjoy the experience of the country. John James Audubon lived on thirty acres of land adjacent to the new cemetery, and was among the elite of New York to be buried there when he died in 1851. John Jacob Astor was buried there in 1848, as was his son, William Blockhouse Astor; the cemetery was to be a place for New Yorkers of the highest station, a manicured landscape of contemplation and rest, removed from the chaos of downtown.[19]

But the distance between the downtown church and the uptown burial ground proved problematic, and the corpses and the landscape in which they rested remained stubbornly difficult to domesticate. By 1862, the vestry was receiving frequent complaints about the state of the grounds, the graves, and the gravestones. The superintendent, it turned out, was a drunk, and the cemetery was a mess. When a committee from the church was finally able to organize a trip to the distant cemetery, the members were shocked by what they found. "Its present aspect is one which may be described as shabby, dilapidated and neglected," the committee reported. "There is no evidence of sufficient care and proper oversight; nor of that affectionate and tender interest with which the sleeping places of the Departed should be kept."[20] The hard work of maintaining a pastoral landscape for the dead had not been done.

A large dog and a bunch of chickens roamed the grounds, rusty pie tins and other garbage was strewn about, and most disgusting, in their opinion, there was "in open view, the skull of a horse, bleached by exposure to the elements." The material evidence of death and decay was upsetting, a jarring reminder of what was happening beneath the soil. And nature itself was getting out of control: trees had not been trimmed, paths were obstructed by overgrown bushes, and plantings on graves had not been tended to. The corpses were being mismanaged, as well: many graves were identified only by a small stick, which could be easily kicked out of the way. Worse still, the church committee found bodies piled in coffins in the receiving vault, some having been there waiting for burial for seven years.[21]

The church leaders discovered that maintaining a pastoral landscape on the city's edge, even after the ideal parcel of land had been secured, would require more careful management and oversight, and would be more expensive than they had expected. Disposal of corpses was hard labor, as was integrating them into a manicured landscape fit for family excursions. It was no easy feat to turn corpses into daisies, and more professional help was required. The "unfit and incompetent," hard-drinking superintendent was fired, and the vestry hired a new superintendent and restructured the way he was supervised. More significantly, they also hired an engineer and a landscape architect to transform the cemetery into a properly picturesque place of rest, and they began plans to irrigate the land, to be certain that plantings could receive proper care through the hot summer months.[22]

Nonetheless, as the city continued to expand toward the cemetery, management became more and more difficult. In 1879, two armed watchmen were added to the cemetery's permanent payroll, and water closets were installed in the public buildings on the grounds.[23] By 1884, there was a new nuisance encroaching on the cemetery: a bathing house on the river within sight of some of the graves. The vestry directed its lawyer to be sure the parties involved did not get the necessary permits from the city. Next, bicycles became a problem, as riders zipping along the cemetery paths disrupted mourners in their peaceful contemplation. New signs were authorized for the cemetery entrances, forbidding use of the machines.[24] As the expanding city encroached on Trinity Church Cemetery, its roles as park and as place of final rest were coming into conflict. A space that had long been available only to the elite of Trinity Church who could afford the long journey north on the island was becoming more and more accessible. The church struggled to manage its cemetery as a private space, but it became ever more difficult to exclude the public from the manicured paths and shaded walks as the city grew up around them.

And the crowding was not just from the outside: the burial plots were filling up, too. By the early twentieth century, it was beginning to become a challenge to find space for all who wanted to be laid to rest there. Regulations on access to the plots became more strict, and in 1929, a columbarium was opened in the cemetery chapel to accommodate ashes of cremated church members.[25]

The Trinity Church Cemetery, once a modest churchyard burial place, was now a sprawling park with engineers, armed guards, administrators, with professional landscaping, complicated record-keeping systems, and storage regimens for handling large numbers of bodies in coffins and bodies in urns. It still maintained its veneer of pastoral simplicity, but the complexity of managing many acres and thousands of bodies in a rapidly urbanizing section of the city more frequently exposed the image for the illusion it was. The cemetery operation was becoming as much factory as park.

The processing of bodies before they reached the cemetery was changing as the city grew, as well. Modest family undertaking businesses had long intermingled with residences in American cities, providing neighborhood families with caskets and hearses and assisting with preparations for funerals. After embalming techniques were advanced during the Civil War, many undertakers added that service to their offerings, allowing families to delay viewings and funerals until distant friends and relatives had arrived for the services, and allowing the shipping of bodies over much longer distances than had previously been practicable.[26]

As the work became more complicated, and as departments of health began requiring more formal permitting and licensing procedures, the businesses became more professional, more concentrated, and more exclusive, and the undertakers who successfully navigated the changes began to do a more brisk trade. The business of handling corpses began to seem more industrial processing than pastoral care, and neighbors were not pleased. Increased traffic of both bodies and mourners, the use of new chemical procedures, and disturbing new processes of handling the corpses made this new funeral industry a nuisance.

Early courts disagreed: a funeral home was not a nuisance per se, though if managed poorly it could become one. In an 1877 decision that was frequently cited throughout the country in later years, the New Jersey Court of Chancery ruled against Ebenezer Westcott, a seventy-two-year-old man trying to stop his undertaker neighbor, Frank Middleton, from plying his trade. Westcott was simply too sensitive, not to noxious fumes or to dangerous chemicals or to disease, but to the mere idea of death. What bothered Westcott was not the way that Middleton conducted his business, but rather the constant reminder of death that the business presented. "Physical discomfort arising from a morbid taste or excited imagination," reasoned the court, "as distinguished from such discomfort arising through the organs of sense common to all, is not sufficient to warrant public or private interference in the conduct of such a lawful business as is the funeral director's profession."[27] Westcott was troubled by the thought of death, and the legal system offered no remedy for troubled thoughts.

The court insisted that there was nothing inherent in the business of running a funeral home that should require its location away from residential areas, drawing a parallel between the work of undertakers and others in the city who deal in perishable wares: just as a grocer might let his vegetables rot out back, or a butcher might let meat grow rancid on the street, an undertaker might conduct his business in such a way as to become a nuisance. "But," the court concluded, "because these things are possible, or may occasionally happen, it is not pretended for a moment that it is unlawful to carry on the grocery business, or to vend meats in the populous parts of our cities. It seems to me that the same reasoning may be applied, with great certainty, to the business of undertaking."[28]

Three decades later, things had changed. In 1910, the Washington Supreme Court argued that urban growth had undercut the reasoning in *Westcott v. Middleton.* As cities were getting larger, and more dense, the justices maintained, it was becoming less appropriate for funeral homes to be located in residential areas. "[I]n this age, when population is becoming more and more congested in the cities, it would be manifestly unfair to grant injunctive relief only in those cases where the object attacked was a nuisance per se, when other circumstances or conditions intervene which might tend to destroy the repose and comfort of a part of a city or town given over to homes," argued the court.[29]

The problem, the court explained, was not so much that a funeral home was dangerous in and of itself, but that morbid thoughts really could be, and that the constant coming and going of dead bodies and funeral processions at a business next door was more than a person could bear. It was common knowledge, the decision stated, "that the immediate presence of those mute reminders of mortality, the hearse, the chapel, the taking in and carrying out of bodies, the knowledge that within a few feet of the windows of one's dwelling-house, where the family sleep and eat and spend their leisure time, autopsies are going on, that the dead are there, cannot help but have a depressing effect upon the mind of the average person, weakening, as the testimony shows, his physical resistance, and rendering him more susceptible to contagion and disease." The mere thought of the relentlessly unending parade of dead bodies through a busy urban funeral home was enough to make a person sick.[30]

Just as twentieth-century dead bodies seemed to be invading peoples' homes and disrupting their repose, urban life was encroaching ever more on the resting places of the dead. In the spring of 1937, Trinity Church closed and locked the public gates to its cemetery for a full year, after "considerable damage was done by persons unknown." The locks didn't solve the problem, though; over the next decade, there was frequent trouble with groups of boys and girls vandalizing gravestones, scaring mourners, and breaking windows in the cemetery buildings. The superintendent was at a loss, reporting in 1942 that "every window in his house had been broken at one time or another." The next decade saw increasing trouble with violence and vandalism at the cemetery, and the problem wasn't solved in 1953, when additional lighting was installed, and safe, well-lit, guarded parking areas were put in place for those visiting the cemetery between 7 and 11 p.m.[31] The pastoral was requiring even more infrastructure and service to maintain.

During the 1970s, the cemetery was not only struggling to preserve its pastoral image in the densely settled neighborhood, but it was almost entirely out of space. By 1975, it was the last active cemetery in Manhattan, and it had only forty-two plots left to sell. This was a serious problem, not only because church members were demanding access to Manhattan resting places for their bodies, but also because the church was committed to perpetual care for the thousands of existing graves, and with no new space for bodies, the cemetery had no source of income to pay for maintenance.[32]

Cremation was seen as the perfect solution. A consultant reported to the vestry in 1975 that the thirty cemeteries serving Manhattan, some of which were forty miles from Times Square, were on average using their last 5 percent of space. The consultant reported that despite the fact that about eighty thousand people a year died in Manhattan, about eight thousand of whom were cremated, no crematories were located on the island. And, he added, the storage potential for ashes—both at the cemetery in Harlem and in niches that could be constructed at the church downtown—was "unlimited." A crematory and storage space for ashes could not only keep the cemetery a revenue-positive operation, but could ultimately generate enough income to sufficiently endow the perpetual care of the graves. "The real profit in the cremation process comes from the sale of niches and urns, or burial space, cremation vault, urn and memorial," the consultant explained. The crematorium itself was merely the processing plant that allowed the sale of less and less space for a corpse.[33]

Since cremation first gained popular acceptance in the United States in the late nineteenth century, advocates have promoted it as a cleaner, more sanitary form of body disposal than burial. Rather than taking up valuable land with an expensive coffin and a rotting body, rather than going through the expensive and chemical-laden process of embalming, a corpse can be reduced to ash and disposed of cleanly and with ease. In truth, however, as with many environmental stories, the process is not so pure as it seems at first.[34]

Cremation ash is legally treated as dirt, as purified dust. With few (and rarely enforced) exceptions, and unlike bodies before burning, there are no regulations as to what can be done with ashes. A body may not be thrown off a bridge, set out in a vegetable garden, kept in a container by the fireplace, but ashes can. Once the body is purified, sterilized, and reduced by extreme heat, it is legally treated as environmentally inert.

However, while people generally imagine that what emerges from a crematorium is a fine, pure, uniform dust, it is in fact more of a gritty meal. Large portions of bone and metal are generally part of the mix, as are teeth. After the corpse is reduced to this jumble of parts by heat and flame, crematoria workers often grind the pieces down, so that the ash is more uniform and more closely resembles the fine dust that people expect. Mixed in with the bone dust, which on its own would be gray, yellow, or white, there is often brown ash from a coffin burned with the corpse. Metal pieces of coffins, copper and gold from jewelry, dental fillings, and metal medical implants are also frequently mixed in. The "cremains," as they are known in the industry, are by no means "pure" or for that matter "natural."[35]

All of which brings us back to the 1991 protests in Harlem. Although the protesters were worried about the burning of pacemaker batteries in corpses, and in particular the plutonium that is part of many of those machines, that particular problem was infrequent by the early 1990s. In the seventies and eighties, there had been frequent and frequently disastrous cases of bodies exploding in crematoria as their pacemakers caught fire. But in the early eighties, New York State (among others) passed a law requiring that bodies delivered to crematoria be certified as battery free. Concerns about elevated mercury levels near crematoria (from the burning of dental fillings) and higher levels of heavy metals (from cancer chemotherapy), as well as toxic smoke from the burning of varnished coffins, seemed cause for legitimate alarm.[36]

The move toward cremation in Harlem was not an environmental improvement for the neighborhood. Rather, it was a way to pack still more bodies onto a crowded piece of land, this time with toxic waste and fumes. With the arrival of the crematorium, it was no longer possible to imagine Manhattan body disposal as pastoral at all; it was a fully industrial process. There were too many bodies, and the bodies themselves had become part of the industrial world.

But where so many efforts to combat the unequal distribution of environmental hazards in Manhattan have been unsuccessful, this protest worked, in part because of the strange power of the idea of the corpse. Polluting a neighborhood with burning flesh could not go on. There are now no crematoria in Manhattan; if you want your ashes to be interred on the island, your body will first be processed in New Jersey.

Notes

This essay is an early exploration of themes and ideas that I am pursuing as part of a book-length project, tentatively titled *Dead as Dirt: An Environmental History of the Dead Body.* For their helpful criticism of earlier drafts of this piece, I would like to thank Ari Kelman, Anne Trubek, Martha S. Jones, John Carson, Christopher Capozzola, Andrew Isenberg, the participants of the Shelby Cullom Davis Center "Nature of Cities" conference at Princeton in December 2003, my fellow fellows at Harvard's Charles Warren Center for Studies in American History (especially Eric Avila), and all of the participants in the center's 2004–5 seminar on the culture and politics of the built environment. I am also grateful to Gregg Mitman and Christopher Sellers for encouraging me to pursue the line of research that led to my initial discovery of the crematorium protests, and to Oberlin College, the American Council for Learned Societies, and the Charles Warren Center for their financial and institutional support of the larger project of which this is a part.

1. Letter from Michel Gelobter, Director of the Office of Environmental Quality, New York City Department of Environmental Protection, to "Elected Official," 19 February 1991; letter from Alfonso R. Lopez, Deputy Director of Facilities Operations, Bureau of Clean Water, New York City Department of Environmental Protection, to "Civic Leader/Concerned Citizen," 5 October 1992; both New York City Municipal Archives Records, Collection 96-15, Box 17, North River Treatment Plant Folder. See also Connie Y. Chiang, "Monterey-By-The-Smell: Odors and Social Conflict on the California Coastline," *Pacific Historical Review* 73, no. 2 (2004): 183–214, for an exploration of the possibilities that odor history presents for environmental historians.

2. Letter from Michel Gelobter, Director of the Office of Environmental Quality, New York City Department of Environmental Protection, to "Elected Official," 19 February 1991; letter from Alfonso R. Lopez, Deputy Director of Facilities Operations, Bureau of Clean Water, New York City Department of Environmental Protection, to "Civic Leader/Concerned Citizen," 5 October 1992; both New York City

Municipal Archives Records, Collection 96-15, Box 17, North River Treatment Plant Folder.

3. E. R. Shipp, "People's Defender Retains a Taste for New Causes," *New York Times,* 19 August 1991, p. B1; Carol Amoruso, "WE ACT for Environmental Justice," *Third Force,* 31 December 1997, p. 19; Nick Ravo, "Residents Say Sewage Is Not the Only Smell," *New York Times,* 18 August 1991, p. A32.

4. Ravo, "Residents Say Sewage Is Not the Only Smell"; Rick Hampson, "The Video That Closed a Crematorium," Associated Press, 1 November 1991.

5. See, for example, Michael Sappol, *A Traffic of Dead Bodies: Anatomy and Embodied Social History in Nineteenth-Century America* (Princeton, N.J.: Princeton University Press, 2002); Gary Laderman, *Rest in Peace: A Cultural History of Death and the Funeral Home in Twentieth-Century America* (New York: Oxford University Press, 2003); Karla F. C. Holloway, *Passed On: African American Mourning Stories* (Durham, N.C.: Duke University Press, 2002); Peter C. Jupp and Glennys Howarth, eds., *The Changing Face of Death: Historical Accounts of Death and Disposal* (London: Macmillan, 1997); Philippe Ariès, *Western Attitudes toward Death: From the Middle Ages to the Present,* trans. Patricia M. Ranum (Baltimore: Johns Hopkins University Press, 1974).

6. Tony Walter, *The Revival of Death* (New York: Routledge, 1994), p. 2.

7. Christopher Sellers, "Thoreau's Body: Towards an Embodied Environmental History," *Environmental History* 4, no. 4 (1999): 486–514; Conevery Bolton Valencius, *The Health of the Country: How American Settlers Understood Themselves and Their Land,* 1st ed. (New York: Basic Books, 2002); Linda Nash, "Finishing Nature: Harmonizing Bodies and Environments in Late Nineteenth-Century California," *Environmental History* 8, no. 1 (2003): 25–52.

8. Nancy Langston, "Gender Transformed: Endocrine Disruptors in the Environment," in *Seeing Nature through Gender,* ed. Virginia Scharff (Lawrence: University Press of Kansas, 2003), pp. 129–66. Another recent work which approaches a more material environmental history of the body is Gerald E. Markowitz and David Rosner, *Deceit and Denial: The Deadly Politics of Industrial Pollution,* California/Milbank Books on Health and the Public, 6 (Berkeley: University of California Press; Milbank Memorial Fund, 2002).

9. Ravo, "Residents Say Sewage Is Not the Only Smell."

10. "Join the Protest Mass March and Rally," (flyer), New York City Community Board Nine Records, September 1991, Community Board Nine offices, Harlem; letter from New York State Senator Franz S. Leichter to constituents, 18 September 1991, New York City Community Board Nine Records, October 1991; "Trinity Crematorium Burns Out in Harlem," *Crain's New York Business,* 2 October 1991, clipping from the "Cemeteries" Vertical File, New York City Municipal Reference Library.

11. "Trinity Crematorium Burns Out in Harlem."

12. Ravo, "Residents Say Sewage Is Not the Only Smell"; Hampson, "The Video That Closed a Crematorium."

13. Warren E. Leary, "Not Even Death Ends Anti-Pollution Crusade," *New York Times,* 27 August 1991, p. C4; "Dangerous When Dead," *Newsweek,* 27 August 1990, p. 56; Stephen Allen, "Mercury 'Danger' in Corpses' Teeth," *The Independent* (London), 16 August 1990, p. 4.

14. Carol Amoruso, "WE ACT for Environmental Justice," *Third Force,* 31 December 1997, p. 19.

15. Percival E. Jackson, *The Law of Cadavers and of Burial and Burial Places,* 2d ed. (New York: Prentice-Hall, 1950), p. 17.

16. Trinity Church Vestry Minutes, Volume III, 1826–50, p. 218, Trinity Church Archives.

17. Howard P. Chudacoff and Judith E. Smith, *The Evolution of American Urban Society,* 3d ed. (Englewood Cliffs, N.J.: Prentice Hall, 1988), p. 89; Roy Rosenzweig and Elizabeth Blackmar, *The Park and the People: A History of Central Park* (Ithaca, N.Y.: Cornell University Press, 1992), p. 5.

18. Trinity Church Vestry Minutes, Volume III, 1826–50, pp. 315–18.

19. David Charles Sloane, *The Last Great Necessity: Cemeteries in American History, Creating the North American Landscape* (Baltimore: Johns Hopkins University Press, 1991), pp. 60–62; Robert B. Dickerson, *Final Placement: A Guide to the Deaths, Funerals, and Burials of Notable Americans* (Algonac, Mich.: Reference Publications Inc., 1982), p. 8; *Churchyards of Trinity Parish in the City of New York, 1697–1969* (New York: The Corporation of Trinity Church, 1948, 1955, 1969), pp. 81, 85, 93.

20. Trinity Church Vestry Minutes, Volume IV, 1850–61, pp. 85, 94; Volume V, 1861–78, pp. 12, 67–70.

21. Trinity Church Vestry Minutes, Volume V, 1861–78, pp. 12, 67–70.

22. Ibid., pp. 12, 71–73.

23. Trinity Church Vestry Minutes, Volume VII, no dates given for volume, pp. 24, 45.

24. Minutes of the Cemetery Committee, 31 May 1884, 2 June 1897, Trinity Church Archives.

25. Minutes of the Cemetery Committee, 5 February 1929. Tax law encouraged the church to merely "lend" the columbarium spaces to members, for a twenty-five-dollar "donation." The members were guaranteed no permanency in the spaces, because to do so would have complicated "ownership" of the chapel, and therefore the tax-exempt status of the church.

26. Gary Laderman, *The Sacred Remains: American Attitudes toward Death, 1799–1883* (New Haven, Conn.: Yale University Press, 1996), pp. 164–75.

27. Arthur Leonard Howell Street, *American Funeral Law: A Manual of Law Affecting Funeral Directors and Embalmers* (Chicago: Trade Periodical Co., 1924), p. 13. *Westcott v. Middleton* (No number in original), Court of Chancery of New Jersey, 43 N.J. Eq. 478; 11 A. 490; 1887 N.J. Super. LEXIS 213, October 1887, Decided.

28. Ibid.

29. *Densmore v. Evergreen Camp, Woodmen of World,* No. 8962, Supreme Court of Washington, Department Two, 61 Wash. 230; 112 P. 255; 1910 Wash. LEXIS 1320, 15 December 1910.

30. Street, *American Funeral Law,* p. 14.

31. Minutes of the Cemetery Committee, 11 April 1938, 20 April 1942, 8 October 1942, 7 November 1946, 10 November 1949, 25 September 1953, 25 February 1954.

32. Memo from Camp Mason to Dr. Robert Ray Parks, 14 November 1975; "Report on the Cemeteries of Trinity Parish, New York City, June 28, 1974," p. 6; both Trinity Church Archives.

33. Memo from Camp Mason to Dr. Robert Ray Parks, 14 November 1975, Trinity Church Archives.

34. See Stephen R. Prothero, *Purified by Fire: A History of Cremation in America* (Berkeley: University of California Press, 2001).

35. Kenneth V. Iserson, *Death to Dust: What Happens to Dead Bodies?* 2d ed. (Tucson, Ariz.: Galen Press, 2001), pp. 291, 322–24.

36. *McKinney's Session Laws of New York,* 204th Regular Session, 1981, Chapter 903; Camillo Fracassini, "Blasted are the Pacemakers," *Scotland on Sunday,* 19 May 2002, p. 14; David Rider, "How Cremation is Supposed to Work," *Ottawa Citizen,* 21 February 2002, p. A10; "Cremation Warning," *New York Times,* 1 November 1981, p. NJ4; Leary, "Not Even Death Ends Anti-Pollution Crusade." Ravo, "Residents Say Sewage Is Not the Only Smell"; "Dangerous When Dead"; "Mercury 'Danger' in Corpses' Teeth."

Part II

The Geography of Power and Consumption

5

Friend or Flood?

The Dilemmas of Water Management in Early Modern Venice

Karl Appuhn

In December 1691, the engineer Matteo Alberti appeared before the Council of Ten—the committee in charge of state security for the Republic of Venice—with a bold proposal.[1] Although Alberti was a Venetian by birth, he had spent much of his adult life abroad. Most recently he had been living in France and the Low Countries where he had studied architecture and learned Dutch flood control and land reclamation techniques.[2] He had returned to his native Venice in the hopes of making his fortune by convincing the leaders of the Venetian Republic to adopt Dutch levee technology to reduce the effects of seasonal floods on the lagoon. Alberti's timing was propitious. In the five years leading up to his appearance before the Council of Ten, Venice and its lagoon had been subjected to a series of increasingly damaging fall and winter floods; and the state was concerned about the mounting expenses associated with repairing the damage wrought by the rising sea waters. Anxious to reduce both the effects of the floods and the expense of maintaining the breakwaters that protected the lagoon, the Republic's leaders were willing to listen to anyone claiming to possess a solution, no matter how improbable; and of all the proposals they heard, Alberti's may have appeared to be the most improbable to Venetian eyes.

The Venetians were no strangers to water management and its associated technologies. Ever since the late thirteenth century, they had deliberately been modifying the lagoon in an ongoing attempt to make it better suit the needs of the city and its port. Indeed, the seasonal flooding episodes that had prompted the Council of Ten to seek the expertise of Alberti and other self-proclaimed water management experts were in part the consequence of four centuries of nearly uninterrupted human intervention in the lagoon environment.[3] In the course of changing the lagoon from a brackish delta marsh to a tidal wetland, the Venetians had developed a set of technologies aimed at regulating and balancing the flow of alluvial and tidal water into the lagoon in the hopes of minimizing the accumulation of sediment in the shipping channels. To accomplish these goals, the Venetians had employed river diversions to redirect and reduce the flow of fresh water into the lagoon; a variety of dredging techniques to reshape the lagoon floor and direct the tidal flux; levees along the mainland side of the lagoon to prevent alluvial flooding; and an array of breakwaters on the marine littoral of the lagoon to prevent higher fall tides and winter storms from eroding the two narrow barrier islands that marked the boundary between the lagoon and the Adriatic. It was these last structures that had lately proven to be the most fragile and expensive component of the system, and it was these that Alberti was proposing to replace with levees designed in what he described as "l'uso d'Holanda," or "the Dutch style."[4]

Despite a long history of state-sponsored lagoon projects, the Venetians were somewhat idiosyncratic water managers in the wider European context. Most other European states, from the nearby Milanese to the more distant Dutch and English, had directed most of their efforts towards irrigation and reclamation projects, an area of water management in which the Venetians had always shown relatively scant interest. A handful of Venetians had publicly advocated reclamation in the lagoon and neighboring wetlands over the course of the sixteenth and seventeenth centuries, but they had generally been treated dismissively by the Republic's leaders.

The Venetians' relative lack of interest in reclamation, both in the lagoon and on the mainland, was due to several interrelated factors. The first was the fact that unlike most other European states, the Venetian Republic had always considered water to be a common resource to be protected from private interests that ran contrary to the perceived public good. For most of Venice's ruling class the public good in this case was synonymous with preserving the lagoon as a large wetland rather than draining it and transforming it into arable as was being done in other parts of Europe. This conviction was underpinned by the celebrated Venetian maxim that a large lagoon made for a large harbor, and the corollary notion that the lagoon was a special environment that required a unique style of stewardship. As a consequence, the Republic had almost invariably sponsored projects aimed at maximizing the lagoon's surface area, even at the expense of neighboring farmland and forests.[5]

The Venetian style of water management was peculiar for another reason as well. Elsewhere in Europe, engineers such as Cornelius Vermuyden had been touting the supposed benefits of a new science of water management, based on a combination of technical expertise and an intimate knowledge of the laws of nature, since the early seventeenth century. The Venetians, on the other hand, had continued to rely on the knowledge of local experts whose ideas and techniques were strongly rooted in practical experience and a well-established Venetian tradition of lagoon management. These experts, usually referred to as *proti* (literally "practiced ones") were not learned engineers claiming to practice a science based on a deductive knowledge of nature's inner workings. Rather they represent an example of what Pamela Smith has called "vernacular science"; men whose technical mastery was drawn from a deep inductive knowledge of Venice's small corner of the natural world and passed down through hands-on training and oral traditions.[6] In the intellectual world of seventeenth-century Europe, the knowledge and prestige of Venetian *proti* and other practitioners of "vernacular science" was gradually being challenged and replaced by that of new types of learned experts, including engineers and natural philosophers.[7] In most public endeavors, however, the Venetians continued to privilege the inductive practices of the *proti,* because they strongly believed that useful knowledge about the natural world could only be derived from an intimate familiarity with specific local conditions.[8]

To a Venetian audience, then, Alberti's Dutch-style scheme must have seemed at once promising and threatening. Promising, because he estimated that the levees would cost only two-thirds as much as the breakwaters to build and be far more durable as well.[9] Threatening, because Alberti was deliberately presenting himself as an engineer selling a project based, in part, on a body of generalized knowledge about how best to build large structures such as breakwaters, rather than on the knowledge of local conditions and practices favored by the Venetians.

Alberti tried to allay any fears about the foreign origins of his technology by claiming that his design rested on a sound empirical foundation: its main features, he emphasized, were the product of centuries of practical experience in the Low Countries. This argument had its drawbacks, however, since a great deal of the inductive knowledge to which Alberti referred had been gathered in the context of large-scale private reclamation projects. In fact, the more informed members of Alberti's audience, including Carlo Guberni (the *proto* in charge of the breakwaters) would later make explicit reference to this inconvenient fact when challenging the project.[10] Nevertheless, the presentation was sufficiently convincing to overcome any initial objections, and the Council of Ten ordered Guberni to select a stretch of breakwater approximately one hundred meters long for Alberti to rebuild the following summer using his Dutch-style design.

Clearly something had happened to persuade the Republic's notoriously conservative patriciate to consider abandoning a long-established flood control technology in favor of a foreign design of dubious origins. In part it was the fact that the past few flood seasons had been particularly disastrous, forcing the Republic to spend far more than usual to maintain and refit the lagoon's seaward defenses (see figure 1). That the floods happened to coincide with a major war against the Ottoman Empire only served to exacerbate their effect on the Republic's finances. The undeniable sense of crisis alone, however, cannot explain why Alberti's scheme was chosen for a field trial, because the Senate and Council of Ten had recently rejected at least three other proposals whose authors claimed to have developed a better, more cost-effective design for the Venetian breakwaters.[11]

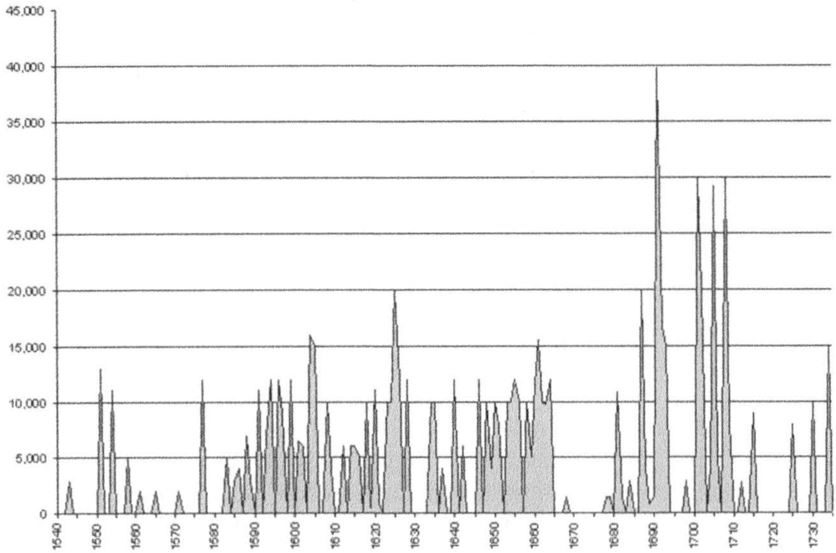

Figure 1. Licenses Issued for Piles Used for the Lido Breakwaters and Levees. This chart shows the number of new oak piles ordered for building and repairing the breakwaters from 1540 to 1735. The lack of consistent narrative sources describing seasonal flooding means that breakwater maintenance provides the best available measure of the gravity of such events. The data were drawn from the *Arsenale, Terminazioni,* and *Senato Terra* series in the Archivio di Stato di Venezia. Note that in 1691 forty thousand new piles were requisitioned, indicating that the autumn of 1690, shortly before Alberti's return to Venice, was the worst in the century and a half since the Venetians had extended the breakwaters. The data also suggest that the severe fiscal crisis that followed the end of the War of Candia in 1669 had led to a period of relative neglect that may have contributed to the devastating flood seasons of the late 1680s. A similar pattern can be seen following the second War of Morea in 1718, and may have helped convince the Senate to adopt Zendrini's plan for permanent stone breakwaters.

Several additional factors probably contributed to the initial success of Alberti's petition. The most important was that the formal training he had received overseas resulted in what was probably the most impressive and unusual presentation the members of the Council of Ten had ever seen. His proposal included a schematic drawing of the proposed structure and a detailed explanation of the principles that underpinned the design. His competitors' proposals, by contrast, were mere elaborations of the standard Venetian breakwater that did not include drawings, and offered little or no explanation of the relative advantages of their designs with respect to the existing structures on the littoral islands. Another important consideration seems to have been the fact that Alberti enjoyed influential connections in the Ducal Palace in the autumn of 1691, in particular his association with Vincenzo Coronelli, Venice's official cartographer and "cosmographer." This connection almost certainly helped him get a hearing and probably added weight to his arguments in the eyes of his audience. Taking into account both of these factors, however, it still remains somewhat surprising that the Council of Ten was willing to devote a substantial amount of capital, labor, and time to a risky proposal based on alien ideas about water management.

This essay will explore the question of why, at the close of the seventeenth century, the Venetians were concerned enough about the problem of seasonal flooding in the lagoon to consider abandoning their traditional reliance on the "vernacular science" practiced by the *proti* in favor of a northern European technology that had been developed to serve a different purpose in a different environmental context. The answer is not merely, as Alberti argued in his first appearance before the Council of Ten, that one design was clearly cheaper and more efficient than the other—the results of the controversial field trial were inconclusive on both counts. Rather, the problem of choosing a breakwater design called into question long-standing Venetian debates over the ideal form of the lagoon and the city; conflicting ideas about what sort of expertise ought to guide lagoon management policies; and deeply rooted attitudes concerning the relationship between humans and nature as mediated through technologies of environmental control.

Matteo Alberti did not openly express an opinion on the broader question of the ideal form of the lagoon and the city in his proposal. Nonetheless, as a Venetian with an interest in both water management and architecture, he could not have been unaware of the fact that the lagoon lay at the very heart of some of the most fiercely contested political debates in Venetian history. Among the more contentious issues was whether the Republic's most important interests lay on the Italian peninsula or with the port and its connections to the larger Mediterranean world. The implications of the choice went beyond economic priorities, evoking the "opposition between a now mythical Venice that derived its wealth and virtue exclusively from the sea, and a Venice that . . . had allowed itself to be drawn in by the temptations of the mainland."[12] Within the context of this larger debate, problems with the lagoon, including flooding and sedimentary accumulation, had often been associated with the alleged corruption that had accompanied the decline of maritime commerce during the sixteenth and seventeenth centuries. The Venetians' sense of themselves as a maritime people and of their city as a commercial capital, therefore, provided a powerful impetus for preserving the lagoon as a large coastal wetland rather than reclaiming its extensive marshy periphery.

The connection between preserving the lagoon and preserving the Republic also extended to the practices and technologies of lagoon management that had been developed by the *proti* over the centuries. As the guardians of the lagoon, they were not merely protecting the harbor, they were protecting the very source of Venetian liberty and virtue; and attacking their actions was seen by many Venetians as tantamount to assaulting the Republic. Thus anyone who wished to challenge their power and expertise had to be careful to do so in a manner that did not raise the specter of the terrestrialization of the lagoon or its residents. Alberti clearly believed that the devastating floods of the previous decade had provided him with an opportunity to do just that, by focusing on the cost-efficiency of traditional Venetian technologies without criticizing their underlying purpose. However, Alberti's challenge, if successful, still had the potential to undermine the traditional large lagoon policy. By replacing the "vernacular science" of the *proti* that had always protected the integrity of the lagoon with a foreign form of expertise that had so often been used to justify large-scale reclamation projects, Alberti would implicitly be opening the door to the idea of converting at least some of the marshy periphery to agrarian uses. Whatever Alberti's intentions, therefore, his proposal was potentially explosive.

THE VENETIAN WATER MANAGEMENT TRADITION

The Venetian tradition of lagoon management went back at least to the eleventh century, and from the outset was inextricably linked to the problem of building and maintaining a city in such an unpromising location.[13] As the urban fabric of the city that would become Venice began to be stitched together, its inhabitants faced two major challenges posed by the difficult delta environment. First there was the problem of building permanent structures on a mudflat, which could only be overcome by driving millions of wooden piles into the soft earth to create stable foundations. Second, and most important for the future of lagoon management, encroaching sediment threatened to block the access to the sea through the three port mouths at San Nicolò, Malamocco, and Chioggia. The Venetians responded by undertaking nearly constant dredging operations in the lagoon, removing accumulated sediment from the lagoon floor and dumping it in the areas of human habitation to create new surface on which to build—a remarkably difficult procedure that often had to be done in the dry.[14]

As Venice became the Mediterranean's most important commercial entrepôt in the high Middle Ages, these two concerns became increasingly urgent. The higher volume of shipping, along with the increasing draft of the ships themselves, meant that maintaining access to the sea was both more important and more difficult. The increasing wealth of the city also meant that larger buildings were being built, with the consequence that new surface area was constantly in demand. The Venice we see today is mostly built on medieval landfill, a process that conditioned the organization of its unique urban space into hundreds of small islands separated by narrow artificial canals.[15]

Eventually, even the expansion of landfill could not keep up with sedimentation, forcing the Venetians to undertake a series of public works designed to alter the lagoon. The projects occurred in two overlapping phases. The first phase—running from the late thirteenth to the mid-seventeenth century—primarily involved river diversions designed to reduce the flow of fresh water carrying large sediment loads into the lagoon. The second phase—running from the early sixteenth to the end of the eighteenth century—involved the construction of breakwaters on the barrier islands to reduce marine erosion and flood damage; and of levees on the mainland periphery of the lagoon to prevent the newly diverted rivers from breaking their banks on the lagoon side of their new beds.

While the two sets of projects may have appeared quite different in concept and intent, at least two common threads held them together. First, they emerged from an empirical tradition of lagoon management that was not much concerned with the world beyond the watershed that fed the lagoon. Most of the theories concerning the effects of alluvial and tidal flows in the lagoon emerged from the efforts to preserve it and, therefore, tended to support the already established parameters for the effort. The first generally recognized theoretical treatise on the lagoon dates from 1442, nearly a century and half after the first river mouths in the southern lagoon were closed, and the subsequent literature remained sparse until the eighteenth century.[16] Moreover, even in the eighteenth century, the Venetians who speculated about the natural history of the lagoon were never concerned with discovering a set of laws that could be used to understand all wetlands; they were concerned exclusively with the problems and prospects of their own lagoon. Thus the Venetians did not develop their management scheme according to a master plan based on a body of deductive knowledge about similar bodies of water. Rather, they proceeded in irregular stages. They would move a river mouth or build a levee, observe the effects of their actions on the lagoon, and then decide whether to pursue further modifications, leave things as they were, or tear the new structures down and start over. This resulted in a number of false starts and reversals of policy. River mouths that had been closed were sometimes reopened if the effects were not judged to be desirable; levees were built, torn down, and built again, depending on the perceived effects on the lagoon.

The second common thread between river diversions and breakwater construction was that they shared a single, clearly understood purpose: to achieve an ideal balance of water and sediment in the lagoon. While occasional disagreements might arise concerning which river mouth to close, or which area of the mainland littoral to dike, the majority of Venetian patricians understood that the goal of all lagoon management projects was to achieve a state wherein the backwater that rushed out of the marshy periphery with the ebb tide would remove the accumulated sediment in the area surrounding the city. Ideally, the lagoon would then become a self-regulating body, no longer requiring active human intervention in the form of dredging and levee building to keep the harbor clear. In practice, the Venetians understood that such a balance could never be struck; but most believed that the concept provided an effective guide for judging the outcome of any given infrastructure project. Thus the ideal of the self-regulating harbor reinforced the empiricism of the Venetian approach to lagoon management by providing a universally agreed-upon measure for the success of any given project.

The Venetian approach to the problem of lagoon management also set up a very specific dynamic between human artifice and nature. As an anonymous author put it in 1413, the goal of human intervention in the lagoon was "to imitate nature."[17] The idea that nature had been intended as a model for humans to follow was quite common in the Renaissance—it was employed by thinkers as diverse as Dante and Copernicus, and informed much of the art of the period—but for the Venetians it had a very specific meaning. The 1413 anonymous represents an early example of a concept of *imitatio naturae* that would be elaborated by later Venetian writers on the lagoon such as Nicolò Contarini. Contarini argued that the lagoon was a fragile and ever-changing environment that normally would not have provided an optimal location for a great city, except that nature had delivered it to its human inhabitants at just the right moment: when its vast extension provided protection from foreign armies and the backwater needed to keep the harbor clear. For the Venetians, therefore, the imitation of nature required that they preserve the lagoon just as it had been given to them by provident nature, not altered to serve the needs of agriculture or left to be swallowed by the sea.[18] The lagoon was understood to be a delicate structure in need of constant care to keep it from being consumed by the dueling forces of earth and sea, and the Venetians were its divinely appointed caretakers.

In the first three centuries of lagoon management, the Venetians were mainly preoccupied with expanding the surface area of the city and altering the flow of fresh water into the lagoon by diverting the three river systems (Piave, Sile, and Brenta) that had originally discharged directly into the lagoon. The results were mixed. While the need for dredging in the harbor was reduced, it was never entirely eliminated. Also, while the accumulation of alluvial sediment in the central lagoon was reduced, the increase in tidal action that resulted from the removal of fresh water flows created new and unexpected difficulties. Sediment continued to accumulate in the *bacino* (the area in front of the Ducal Palace where most ships anchored), much of it brought in by the incoming tide and deposited against the embankments or on the large mudflat next to the island of San Giorgio on the opposite side of the harbor. Whatever its source, however, sediment remained a familiar foe. What the Venetians had not been expecting were the completely novel difficulties caused by their efforts at preserving the lagoon. The increasing salinity of the lagoon, for example, brought with it seasonal seaweed infestations that clogged canals and trapped waste products that were supposed to exit the lagoon on the ebb tide.

The most dramatic consequence of the river diversions was a measurable increase in the period of the tidal flux. Stronger tidal action introduced seasonal flooding into the lagoon environment. The Venetians soon discovered that when higher autumn flood tides coincided with the warm south wind known as the sirocco, the water levels in the lagoon would rise well above normal. Now known as *acqua alta* (high water) the phenomenon of the *siroccali* was well known and understood by the sixteenth century; and while much of the city did not flood as often as it does now, water in the Piazza San Marco—the lowest point in the city—became a regular feature of Venetian life. The patrician Marino Sanudo, whose voluminous diaries cover daily life in Venice in the first thirty-five years of the sixteenth century, makes occasional reference to seasonal floods submerging the city, and dozens of references to water in the Piazza San Marco.[19] He also mentions frequent damage to the outlying settlements of Malamocco and Chioggia caused by higher fall tides.[20] By the early sixteenth century, seasonal flooding had become a regular feature of life in Venice.

Seasonal flooding forced the Venetians to begin modifying their approach to managing the lagoon. River diversions were useful in terms of preventing the terrestrialization of the further reaches of the lagoon, thereby assuring the accumulation of backwater, but the increase in tidal action was having tangibly negative effects on the port. Tidal deposits not only posed a danger to the inner harbor, but they also threatened to block the three entrances to the lagoon at Chioggia, Malamocco, and San Nicolò. To counter the effects of sedimentary accumulation, and to prevent the barrier island settlements from flooding, large breakwaters were erected at the entrances of the lagoon to increase the speed at which water flowed through the channels. The breakwaters were considered remarkable enough that foreign dignitaries sometimes asked to see them as part of their visits to the city.[21] As the floods increased in severity in the first half of the sixteenth century, the breakwaters were gradually extended from the port mouths to protect sections of the two main barrier islands where marine erosion threatened to create new openings to the sea. Eventually the new breakwaters would extend along four kilometers of the island of Pellestrina and about twelve hundred meters of Sottomarina, which, added to the breakwaters at the harbor mouths, gave the Venetians well over six kilometers of exposed breakwater to repair and maintain. By the late sixteenth century, fall floods and winter storms had begun to rise above the level of the islands, washing sediment directly into the lagoon and clogging the channel that led from the port mouth at Malamocco to the *bacino.* By the middle of the seventeenth century, such episodes had become so severe that the accumulation of sediment blocked the Republic's larger warships inside the harbor during the War of Candia (1645–69), forcing the Arsenal's shipbuilders to disassemble the upper decks of the ships in order to move them in and out of the lagoon.[22]

The increasing size and scope of the public works projects led to the bureaucratization of lagoon management. In 1501 a new office, the *savii alle acque,* or water managers, was created to coordinate lagoon management efforts, and to impede the terrestrialization of the lagoon.[23] Four years later a larger body, the *collegio alle acque,* was formed to hear and rule on proposals to modify the lagoon, especially in areas where backwater accumulated. Most of the cases on which the *collegio alle acque* would be called to rule involved reclamation projects along the shores of the lagoon. It was in the early decades of the sixteenth century, then, that the large lagoon policy became articulated in legal terms as a struggle between the desire of individual landowners to enrich themselves and the public good that derived from a functional harbor and the largest possible lagoon. Here again, the Venetian conception of the role played by human artifice in controlling nature helped set the terms of the debate. The public good was best served by preserving the lagoon as nature had intended it, not exploiting it for agrarian purposes. Private interests, in short, were counterproductive when they conflicted with the large lagoon policy.

For most historians of Venice, the struggle between public and private interests in the lagoon is best illustrated by the fierce sixteenth-century polemic between the most famous proponent of private reclamation in the lagoon, Alvise Cornaro, and the most articulate defender of the large lagoon policy, Cristoforo Sabbadino. The Sabbadino-Cornaro polemic occupies a privileged place in the historiography, because it perfectly encapsulates the stakes of the large lagoon policy.[24] Sabbadino, a *proto* in the service of the *savii alle acque,* defended the idea of the large lagoon so vigorously that he is often mistakenly credited with having invented it. His opponent, Alvise Cornaro, explicitly called into question the Venetian notion of *imitatio naturae*—and by extension the large lagoon policy—by attacking the Venetian insistence on devoting such a large area to unproductive tidal flooding.

Cornaro, was, like Matteo Alberti, an expatriate Venetian with a longstanding interest in water management and reclamation. He had abandoned Venice for nearby Padua as a youth, after his claim to patrician status had been rejected by the Great Council.[25] In Padua, Cornaro had dedicated himself to study and agriculture. In a series of pamphlets and treatises, he claimed to have made a considerable fortune by buying up worthless swamp land, draining it, and converting it to cereal production. The endeavor had not only brought him wealth, Cornaro said, but physical health and long life, benefits that could be extended to all members of Venetian society if the Republic would only subsidize large-scale reclamation projects in the lagoon.

Cornaro also published a series of open letters to the Venetian Senate in which he outlined a number of ambitious plans for reshaping the lagoon. His most controversial idea involved building a dike along the mainland littoral and draining the peripheral marshland, leaving Venice as an island in the middle of a large harbor. Cornaro dismissed the idea that the consequent reduction in backwater would have dire consequences for the harbor and the city, observing that most harbors were not attached to large lagoons. In another treatise he advocated turning the lagoon around the city into an artificial lake, cut off from the harbor by a series of dikes. In a third he proposed building a new island featuring a loggia, a sunken theatre, and a giant fountain directly across the *bacino* from the Ducal Palace.

Cornaro's treatises were, in some respects, a form of intellectual play, a way of displaying his considerable learning to his peers. Yet he also intended for them to be taken seriously by the Senate, despite the fact that he was attacking the Venetians' most basic assumptions about how the lagoon should be managed. He was also violating Venetian ideas about the proper source of expertise. In spite of his authoritative pronouncements, Cornaro had no knowledge of the effects of reclamation on the lagoon, and while he had certainly invested in reclamation projects, his actual understanding of the process was limited. As if to emphasize his lack of practical experience, Cornaro adopted the title *architectus,* which was meant to stress his study of classical and contemporary treatises on urban planning and architectural design—he had written a commentary on the Roman architectural writer Vitruvius—but only called attention to the fact that had never built a building.[26]

Cornaro's lack of experience with applied architecture stood in stark contrast to that of his opponent Cristoforo Sabbadino, the chief *proto* in the employ of the *savi alle acque.* Sabbadino mocked Cornaro for his reliance on books, arguing that the only reliable guide to lagoon management was hard-won experience.[27] Sabbadino was not university educated. His father had been a *proto* in the field of water management, and Cristoforo had followed him in the family business—the Sabbadino family would continue to feature prominently as *proti* well into the eighteenth century.

Despite the importance accorded to it by historians, the Sabbadino-Cornaro polemic was no contest. Cornaro was a commercially successful author, and he may have thrilled his readers with the bravura of his humanist-inspired learning; but when it came to making real decisions about lagoon management, the empirical expertise of the *proto* was the only kind of knowledge the Republic's leaders were willing to trust. Cornaro may have motivated individual patricians to pursue reclamation on their own mainland properties, but he did not persuade the Senate to sacrifice backwater in favor of cereal production.

Sabbadino, for his part, is remembered as the chief architect of sixteenth-century urban planning in Venice. He drew up the first integrated plan for lagoon management, which included one of the first attempts to accurately map the lagoon, and authored an ambitious plan of urban expansion in the area known as *fondamenta nuove* that was completed in 1590, thirty years after its author's death.[28] An important part of his legacy was the formalization of the large lagoon policy, and a far more precise interest on the part of the state in understanding and regulating the flow of water in the lagoon. In 1620, the Senate followed up on Sabbadino's mapping efforts with the decision to undertake a vast project to chart precisely the boundaries of the lagoon, including detailed soundings of even the most remote corners of the wetlands. Known as the *conterminazione lagunare,* the project took nearly two centuries to complete, but the principle behind it—the preservation of the boundaries of the lagoon against encroachment by greedy landowners—was as old as the first river diversions.[29]

The *conterminazione* project was only one of many that occupied the Republic's water managers in the century following Sabbadino's death. New, more dramatic river diversions were undertaken by the Republic and its client cities on the mainland. The *savi alle acque* began to look beyond the borders of the lagoon for solutions to the challenges posed by the city's unique environment.[30] Most famously, the Republic attempted to reshape the Adige and Po deltas so that they would discharge their waters to the south, in the hopes of reducing the amount of sediment suspended in the northern Adriatic and pushed into the lagoon with each tidal cycle.[31] It was also in this period that the breakwaters along the barrier islands were extended beyond the areas around the harbor mouths. The undertaking dwarfed the medieval efforts, but it remained grounded in the same set of principles, especially in the notion that a balance between water and sediment that would preserve the ideal form of the lagoon ought constantly to be sought, even if it could never fully be achieved.

In the century following Sabbadino's death the Republic's various water management projects became more integrated in the service of a single program. It was during this process of integration that Venetian projects began to look anomalous by European standards. While Dutch engineers were spreading the gospel of reclamation to England, Germany, and beyond, the Venetians steadfastly adhered to a strategy based on the conservation of coastal wetlands. Several Dutch *dijkmeisters* visited Venice during the seventeenth century, but the main thing the Venetians were interested in getting from them were the plans for better dredging equipment for keeping the main shipping channels clear.[32] Even as the effects of the *siroccali* worsened, and the seventeenth-century European climatic deterioration brought more severe winter storms to batter the breakwaters, flood the city, and deposit sediment in the lagoon, the Venetians remained confident in the idea that their appointed task was to preserve the lagoon as an extensive wetland. That they were never seriously tempted to change course is testimony to how powerfully entrenched the traditional approach to lagoon management had become, and of the degree to which the Republic continued to trust the "vernacular science" of the *proti* over virtually all forms of outside expertise.

ALBERTI'S EXPERIMENT

By the time Alberti returned to his native city in 1691 with the intention of selling the Republic's leaders on the virtues of Dutch water management technology, the Venetian water management tradition, including the reliance on *proti* and the large lagoon policy, had become an unquestioned component of Venetian political culture. Private landowners whose property bordered the lagoon understood that seeking approval for reclamation projects was futile, and resorted to surreptitiously draining adjoining wetlands and trusting in litigation to protect them in case of discovery. No one had mounted a credible attack against Venetian ideas about the lagoon in well over a century.

Alberti could hardly have been unaware of the fact that the he was challenging deeply held beliefs about Venice's place in the world and that he had to proceed cautiously if his bid to become the Republic's first water engineer were to be successful. He was careful, therefore, not to raise any issues that might have recalled the ghosts of Sabbadino and Cornaro, or have brought to mind the possibility that his project might lead to reclamation in any form. He stressed two factors only—cost and durability—while avoiding any discussion of the larger water management context within which the structures he was proposing were meant to function. In this regard, his proposal looks very much like those of other individuals who appeared before the Council of Ten claiming to possess the secret to a better breakwater that could be built on the cheap.

If he tried to make his proposal indistinguishable from those of his competitors in terms of content, Alberti worked hard to make it stand out in terms of form. He took every opportunity to display the fruits of his northern education. He began by conspicuously and repeatedly referring to himself as "ingegnere Matteo Alberti." "Engineer" was a title that was widely employed in northern Europe, but it was little used in Venice—Alberti was among the first to adopt it there. He clearly hoped that the title would convey the kind of practical experience with breakwater construction that his fellow Venetians would be comfortable with, while at the same time connoting the fact that he had received a formal education in the principles of architecture and was a man of science.

Alberti's connection to science and the world of natural philosophy would have been enhanced in the minds of his audience by his close association with Vincenzo Coronelli. The Republic's official "cosmographer" was an encyclopedist and cartographer of considerable fame throughout Europe. He was a favorite of Doge Francesco Morosini due his 1685 publication, *Memorie istoriografiche del regno di Morea e Negroponte,* an atlas of Morosini's recent Peloponnesian conquests. Coronelli was also a high-ranking Franciscan and in 1701 he would be elected minister general of the order. It appears quite likely that Coronelli's influence at the Ducal Palace had gained Alberti his initial audience before the Council of Ten. Like his friend, Coronelli had spent time in northern Europe, including trips to France, the Dutch Republic, and England, where he knew both Edmund Halley and Robert Hooke. Today Coronelli is perhaps best remembered for the pair of globes depicting the earth and the heavens that he built for Louis XIV, but in the late seventeenth century he would have been equally famous as the first encyclopedist to organize the entries of his compendium alphabetically, and as the founder of Europe's first geographic society: the *Accademia degli Argonauti* (Academy of the Argonauts) of which Alberti was a member.[33] At the time of Alberti's appearance before the Council of Ten, Coronelli was busy producing a new work, the *Atlante Veneto,* a universal atlas that was intended to compile all available geographic knowledge in a single series of volumes. To produce the atlas he had sent out thousands of questionnaires to correspondents as far away as North America in hopes of creating maps that included as much verifiable geographical information as possible.

For Coronelli, geography entailed not only the production of maps and globes, but the advancement of all realms of knowledge connected to the earth, including geology.[34] In this sense, Coronelli was more than just an encyclopedist and a mapmaker; he was the most important representative of natural philosophy in Venice at the end of the seventeenth century. Although he did not voice an official opinion concerning Alberti's design for the littoral breakwaters, he clearly shared the engineer's interests in hydrostatics and water management and was considered an authority on the subject outside of Venice. In 1711, following a winter of devastating floods, Coronelli would draw up a proposal for dredging the Adige River; in 1716 he would submit his own proposal for improving the littoral breakwaters; and in 1717 he would leave Venice for Vienna to become the Commissioner and Superintendent of the Danube under Emperor Charles VI.

Alberti, then, was a member of an unusual group in Venice, where the precepts and goals of natural philosophy had not taken root to any great extent. Coronelli and his circle constituted the leading edge of an attempt to get Venetians to embrace natural philosophy and its attendant benefits. Alberti's attempt to replace the management regime of the *proti* with scientifically grounded technologies is best understood as part of this effort, as is his confidence that the universal laws of nature dictated that his design would work just as well in Venice as it had in the Low Countries.

Alberti further bolstered his claims to expertise through a display of his architectural and mathematical training. His proposal included a schematic drawing comparing his design with that of the structures currently in use (see figure 2); an explanation of the principles that made his design more

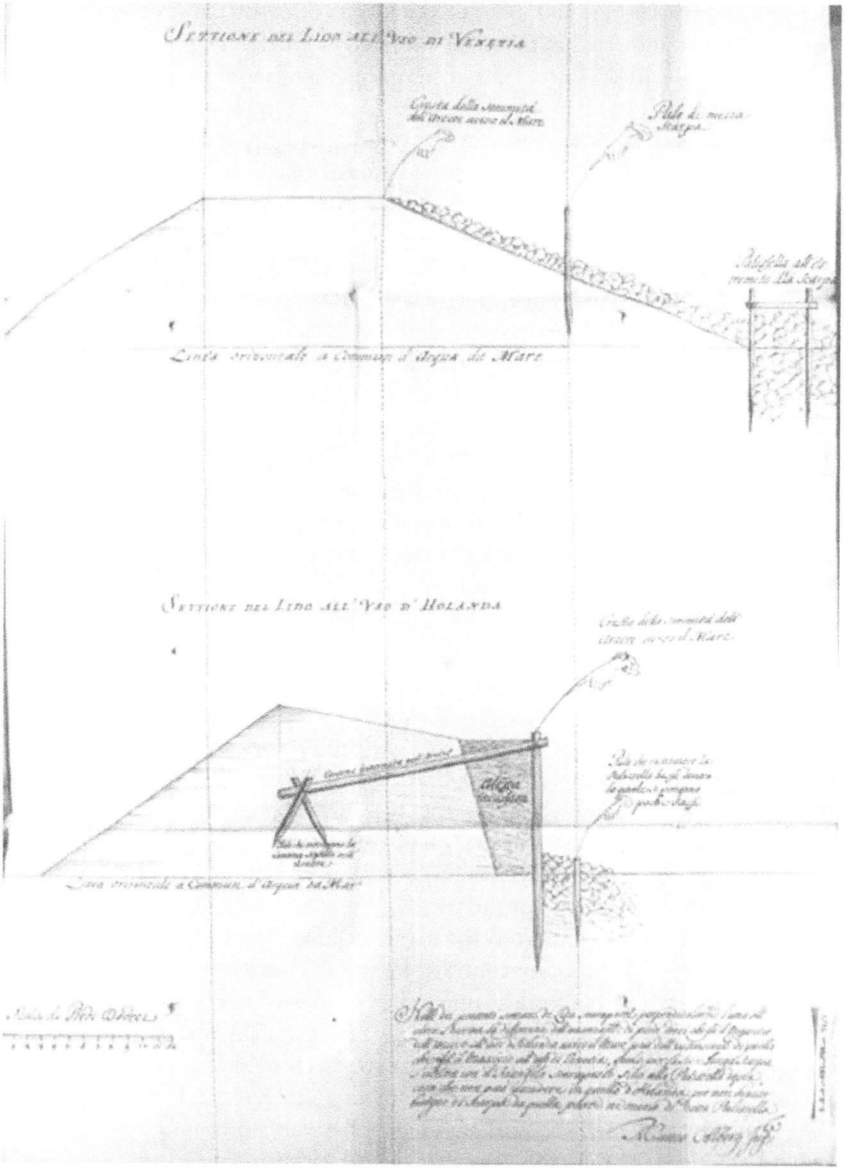

Figure 2. Matteo Alberti's technical drawing comparing the Venetian design (top) with his Dutch-style design (bottom). The long horizontal line represents mean sea level. The scale is in Venetian feet. Note the signature at the bottom right, which reads "Matteo Alberti Ingegnere," as does all of his correspondence with the Council of Ten and the Collegio alle Acque. ASV, Savi ed esecutori alle acque, B. 72, c. 38. Reproduced by permission of the Ministero per i Beni e le Attività Culturali.

durable than the other; and a detailed analysis of construction costs for both structures that showed his to be far more economical. While Venetians had been among the first Europeans to employ topographical maps, and were thus accustomed to the use of visual devices in presentations such as Alberti's, schematic drawings like the one he had produced were extremely unusual—his is the earliest surviving schematic of a breakwater in the Venetian archives—as were his efforts to explain the principles that underpinned the design. Indeed, the sheer amount of detail in his presentation was overwhelming in comparison to the other three that had been submitted to the Council of Ten that year, none of which discussed the structural principles of the design or contained anything resembling a comparative cost analysis.

Alberti expressed no opinion on the subject of the overall management regime in the lagoon. Indeed, he made every effort to suggest that that his design would easily fit into the existing scheme. He stressed that the Dutch technology was the product of both science and centuries of practical experience, and thus presumably more like the traditional Venetian breakwaters than the members of the Council might think. He was careful to avoid any mention of reclamation, despite the fact that the technology he was selling had mostly been used to that end. At every turn he tried to emphasize the compatibility of his technology with the Venetian worldview. Nevertheless, by arguing that a design based on the universal laws of hydrostatics was both more effective and cheaper than the traditional Venetian design, he was challenging the very basis of the *proti*'s expertise: an intimate familiarity with what were presumed to be the unique conditions of the Venetian lagoon.

Most of the differences between Alberti's design and the conventional Venetian breakwater are clear in the technical drawing he provided. The Venetian design featured sloping earthworks supported by a main row of large oak piles and covered with a protective layer of stone. At the base of the earthworks where the wave front struck, the structure was composed of two rows of smaller piles supported by a wall of loose stone in the gap between the rows. Alberti's design, by contrast, featured a near vertical wall facing the sea, and only two rows of piles supporting a smaller stone-filled enclosure at the base of the structure. The other novel features of the design were the horizontal supports attached at intervals to the back of the main pile wall and anchored in the earthworks, and the use of an aggregate made out of seaweed, lime, and crushed earth behind the main pile wall (indicated by the shaded area on the drawing). Finally, the earthworks that supported the breakwater was nearly four feet higher with respect to mean sea level than the Venetian design, a feature that Alberti argued made it better able to withstand the exceptionally big autumn and winter seas that had occasionally topped the Venetian structures in recent years.

In his cost analysis, Alberti argued that his design offered short-term savings due to more efficient use of materials, as well as long-term savings derived from the greater durability of the structures. The main material savings came from a reduction in earth-moving costs. While Alberti's earthworks structure was of similar volume to the Venetian design, about 20 percent of the total volume was composed of the seaweed aggregate, which, he claimed, cost half as much to produce and move as earth brought in on barges from the mainland because all of the material could be collected in the lagoon itself. Also, Alberti's design used only 25 percent as many stones as the Venetian design as there was no sloping earth berm to protect. Acquiring and moving the stones to protect the pile walls was the single most expensive component of the Venetian structures, and it was there that Alberti promised the greatest savings. The one area where his design did not employ fewer materials was in its use of timber. The elimination of one of the pile walls was offset by the need for the anchored supports, although these could be of less expensive material than the oak piles used in the main walls. Finally, Alberti contended that the vertical wall would be better able to withstand the constant assault of the waves, and be less likely to give way and allow the higher autumn floods to wash over the islands and into the lagoon.

The combination of Alberti's personal associations and the quality of his presentation convinced the Council of Ten to grant him a stretch of breakwater on which to experiment with his design; but the Council was easier to impress with statistics and technical drawings than Alberti's next audience, the Venetian official in charge of maintaining the breakwaters: *proto ai lidi* Carlo Guberni.

Guberni did not respond directly to Alberti's plan at the outset, limiting himself to acknowledging the request to find an appropriate stretch of damaged breakwater for Alberti to rebuild. He did not, however, remain mute in the face of this challenge to the basis of his expertise. In May of 1692 he wrote a long letter to his patrician superiors, the *savii alle acque,* in which he indirectly attacked several features of Alberti's proposal by defending the main features of the basic Venetian design. He also took the opportunity to propose some minor alterations of his own, perhaps as a way to remind the *savi* that the *proti* were capable of innovation too.[35] In the letter, Guberni refers to "recent suggestions," a category that included both Alberti's project and the other three petitions offering new breakwater designs. The four proposals in question had contained a number of important changes to the existing design, including raising the overall height of the structures; thinning, shortening, or lengthening the piles; widening or narrowing the base of the earthworks; and in one case, eliminating the protective layer of rock on the front of the berm. Guberni limited himself to attacking the features that the others shared with Alberti's design.

Guberni began by criticizing the idea of raising the height of the earthworks, one of Alberti's strongest arguments in favor of the Dutch technology. He derisively referred to taller structures as "a show for the eyes that serves no purpose," because the real challenge lay beneath the waterline, not at the crown of the structures. He reiterated his point when he dismissed the idea of redistributing the piles closer to the face of the breakwater structure, arguing that because the action of the wave front was constantly eroding the bases of the piles that held the rocks in place, it was necessary to set one line of piles further back. Otherwise, he argued, the piles and rocks could all be pulled loose in a short period of time, allowing the sea to undermine the entire structure and leading inevitably to internal collapse. Shortening the base of the earthworks by creating a steeper slope, Guberni said, would simply make the entire structure more vulnerable to the vicissitudes of tide and storm, because by the time the damage became evident, the main structure would already have been compromised. By contrast, he concluded, the gentle slope of the Venetian design provided advance warning of impending failure as well as the opportunity to make inexpensive repairs rather than being forced to undertake wholesale replacement of the structures every time a section failed.

Instead of focusing on the visible part of the structure, Guberni said, builders needed to consider what was happening at the base. To illustrate his point, Guberni referred the *savi* to the section of breakwater in front of the Church of the Virgin in Chioggia. Recent alterations to the mouth of the Brenta had led to the accumulation of sediment in front of the base of the breakwater, with the result that it had been transformed from one of the least stable sections in the system to one of the most durable. If Venice's leaders were serious about improving the performance of the breakwaters, Guberni concluded, they would be looking at ways to promote the accumulation of sediment along the entire length of the system, not worrying about the height of the structures or the number of piles and rocks they contained. To accomplish this goal, Guberni favored the addition of groins perpendicular to the main structure, but he also suggested sinking decommissioned ships in front of the breakwaters as a more cost-effective alternative for protecting the vulnerable base of the breakwaters.

Despite the fact that he did not once mention Alberti by name, Guberni was clearly addressing himself to the engineer's project. There was no pressing need to respond to any of the other proposed designs, since Alberti's was the only one that had been given a field trial. Moreover, he focused his attacks on the features that the various proposals shared with Alberti's design, especially the raising and shifting of the earthworks closer to the water, while ignoring the minor changes to the basic Venetian design proposed by the other petitioners such as leaving the berm unprotected. Guberni's letter also served as a powerful demonstration of his detailed understanding of the conditions that held on the barrier islands; and by extension showed that he was far better equipped to diagnose the problems with the Venetian breakwaters than someone whose design was based on a general understanding of the laws of nature and the principles of architecture.

By not identifying Alberti and his project by name, Guberni acquired an advantage in the debate to come. When Alberti inevitably tried to claim that Guberni had tried to sabotage his project out of personal enmity or professional jealousy, Guberni could point out that he had never once mentioned Alberti's name in any of his official correspondence. At the same time, his letter was not merely diagnostic, it was predictive. If, as he suspected, Alberti's design did prove vulnerable to erosion beneath the waterline, he could point back to the letter as incontrovertible proof of the superiority of the *proto*'s knowledge over that of the *ingegnere.*

Guberni's strategy proved prescient. By late August of 1692, Alberti was already complaining to the *savi alle acque* that his project was being compromised by delays in the delivery of material—seaweed for the aggregate, oak piles, and rocks for the wall—and by the fact that Guberni had chosen a particularly bad location for the experiment.[36] Receiving no reply, Alberti followed up with a lengthy letter on 1 September, in which he repeated his objection to the site that had been chosen for him on the island of Pellestrina.[37] He complained that before he could begin construction, he would have to clear the site of the debris from the destroyed breakwater, a chore that threatened to set him back at least a week or two. While Alberti acknowledged the need to demonstrate that his design could hold up under the toughest possible conditions, he felt that the impending change of season and the delivery delays entitled him to a simpler site. He then proposed four possible alternatives to the Pellestrina site.

Guberni chose this moment to rise to the challenge and confront Alberti directly. For the first time he mentioned Alberti by name, but instead of acknowledging his expertise by referring to him as *ingegnere,* he pointedly called him "Signor Alberti." He acknowledged that the site was exposed, but he stressed that there were far worse places he might have chosen, naming five examples to reinforce the point. He then estimated that with eight or ten men Alberti could clear the site in three or four days at most. He also criticized Alberti's apparent refusal to reuse materials salvaged from the existing structure, pointing out that it was standard practice to save any piles that had not been consumed by rot or eaten away by worms. He noted that years of practical experience with reusing materials had proven that used piles in good condition lasted just as long as new piles, as they were likely to be washed away well in advance of wearing out. Thus it was Alberti's profligate use of new materials that was causing delays and cost overruns, Guberni argued, not the site.

Guberni also chose this moment to reveal that the cost comparison Alberti had provided with his original proposal had been badly botched. Not only had Alberti failed to take into account the Venetian practice of reusing old materials when refitting sections of breakwater, but he had also distorted the figures to make the difference in costs between the two structures seem far greater than it really was. While pretending to compare the costs per *pertega* (approximately two meters) of breakwater, he had actually compared his cost per *pertega* with the Venetian cost per *passo* (approximately three meters) which meant that the adjusted costs were actually nearly identical, and that no long-term economic advantage would accrue from switching to Alberti's design.

Finally, Guberni defended himself against recent rumors—probably circulated by Alberti—that he was actively trying to sabotage the experiment to preserve his position and protect the illicit gains he made at public expense by skimming off the cost of materials. Guberni pointed out that his family had been serving as *proti ai lidi* for a century now; that his father, grandfather, and uncle had all died destitute after serving in the office; and that if he was able to make a living at all, it was thanks to his maternal inheritance. Indeed, Guberni's own will would seem to confirm his claims. He left two small bequests to local hospitals, endowed six months' worth of masses in his name at the church in Malamocco, asked for the cheapest funeral available, and left his few household furnishings to his concubine and his daughter-in-law.[38] If he had amassed ill-gotten gains from his service to the Republic, they remained well hidden at the time of his death.

Still, Guberni had yet to address the specifics of Alberti's design directly, limiting himself to responding to accusations of malfeasance on his part and pointing out gross errors in the engineer's cost analysis. As Alberti continued to complain that the project was being delayed by missing materials, bad weather, the characteristics of the site, and other causes beyond his control, Guberni resumed his earlier silence, allowing Alberti to undermine his own credibility with increasingly desperate and frustrated letters. It was in one of these letters that Alberti made his first and only reference to the traditional lagoon management scheme. Seething with frustration at Guberni's refusal to respond to his pleas for additional money and manpower, Alberti stated that the *proto* did not understand the advantages of the Dutch design because he did not recognize that the purpose of the breakwaters was to "separate the water of the sea from that of the lagoon through human artifice," rather than encourage the ingress of the sea into the lagoon.[39] Alberti did not pursue this line of argument any further, but it seems clear that he had more in mind than just rebuilding the Venetian breakwaters when he had attacked the Venetian tradition of inductive knowledge about the lagoon. It also suggests that he was perfectly aware that by undermining the credibility of the *proti,* he was calling into question the entire Venetian tradition of lagoon management. Despite having been presented with such an inviting target, Guberni refused to respond. It was only in late December of 1692 that he returned to the fray, finally taking up the technical aspects of Alberti's design.[40] While stating that he would rather leave a commentary on the principles of the design to an architect, he pointed out that Alberti's structures had already suffered damage, casting doubt on their ability to stand up to years of exposure to the elements. He also claimed that part of the problem with the design was due to Alberti's insistence on building it along the same plane as the Venetian structures when it was now clear that it would have worked better to place the face of the breakwater ten feet back, behind the protective cover of the beach. In fact, in the Low Countries, such structures were always protected by a wide strip of sand and dunes, and Guberni was correct in his assumption that the design was not meant to stand up to the direct action of the sea. Of course, since one of the main problems facing the Venetians was beachfront erosion, setting the structures back would only have served to delay the inevitable and further reduce the width of the barrier islands that protected the lagoon.

Guberni then returned to the issue of Alberti's cost analysis, pointing out several more discrepancies. He closed the letter with what was, in the judgment of an empirically trained *proto,* the most damning evidence of all: that Alberti's structures had suffered a great deal of damage, despite the fact that the season had been quite mild, with only the Piazza San Marco flooding in the city itself, and no serious damage reported to the rest of the Venetian breakwaters. Alberti, who had been so vocal throughout the autumn, was finally silent.

Guberni's final report on the matter was filed at the end of March. Accompanied by two other *proti,* Guberni spent a day surveying the season's damage to Alberti's breakwaters.[41] Guberni was able to refer to his predictions of the previous May, and with the confidence of hindsight to use them to attack Alberti's project. Alberti's structure had failed in the very manner Guberni had predicted. Two sections of the front wall had been torn away by the sea, allowing water to enter at the base of the earthworks where it had eaten through the layer of aggregate, washed away soil from inside the structure, and caused the internal collapse of two sections of the main structure. In the end, Guberni observed, the entire earthworks would have to be replaced, mitigating whatever modest savings might have been generated by the engineer's construction techniques.

Guberni's report put an end to Alberti's experiment. The knowledge, both practical and predictive, of the Venetian *proto* had seemingly triumphed over the sophistication of the formally trained engineer and his northern European outlook. This was certainly how Guberni saw it, and the Venetian ruling class appears to have agreed with his assessment. The breakwaters continued to be supervised by *proti* until after the fall of the Republic in 1797, and never again would their expertise be seriously challenged by an outsider. Alberti's thoughts on the matter were not recorded. In the wake of his public humiliation he left Venice for good, and assumed the post of supervisor of fortifications for Johann Wilhelm, the Elector Palatine.

In the decades following the experiment, the Venetians continued to seek a better solution to the problem of marine erosion on the barrier islands. In

1716 Vincenzo Coronelli submitted an anonymous proposal to the Senate for the replacement of the earth and timber structures with new structures composed entirely of stone.[42] Like Alberti, Coronelli included a schematic drawing in support of his proposal. The drawing shows a steeply sloping structure with narrow steps extending into the water and looks very much like a stone version of Alberti's Dutch-style structures. Coronelli, who had since fallen from favor in both Venice and Rome, was not taken seriously by the Senate, nor was he afforded the same opportunity as Alberti to test his structures under actual conditions. When the Senate finally resolved to build a series of permanent stone breakwaters in 1735, Coronelli's design was not even mentioned in passing. The new breakwaters were not the brainchild of an *ingegnere* like Alberti or a natural philosopher like Coronelli. They were designed by a *proto* named Bernardino Zendrini. Begun in 1744, construction on Zendrini's *murazzi* took thirty-eight years to complete. Fourteen meters at the base and one meter at the crown, Zendrini's design was closely modeled on the traditional Venetian earth and timber breakwater it was meant to replace. Even in the transition to stone and concrete barriers, the Venetians stuck with traditional technologies, traditional sources of expertise, and a traditional conception of the relationship between human artifice and the lagoon.

NOTES

I would like to thank Edward Muir, Alfredo Viggiano, Matteo Casini, Kinch Hoekstra, Susan Morrissey, Jonathan Israel, and Noah Efron for their comments on this essay. I would also like to thank the Gladys Krieble Delmas Foundation and the American Philosophical Society, whose financial assistance made the research possible.

1. Archivio di Stato, Venezia (hereafter ASV), Consiglio dei Dieci, Parti Comuni, Filza, Dicembre 1691.

2. *Dizionario biografico degli italiani,* vol. 1 (Rome: Istituto della Enciclopedia Italiano, 1960), pp. 714–15. The entry claims that in 1672 Alberti was involved in another major project involving the littoral breakwaters, but since he would have been twelve years old at the time, this seems a dubious proposition. It would appear more likely that someone mistakenly transcribed the "9" in "1692" as a "7," thus leading to the confusion.

3. See Élisabeth Crouzet-Pavan, *"Sopra le acque salse": Espaces, pouvoir, et société a Venise, a la fin du moyen âge,* 2 vols. (Rome: Istituto Storico Italiano per il Medio Evo, 1992); and John Keahey, *Venice against the Sea: A City Besieged* (New York: St. Martin's Press, 2002).

4. ASV, Consiglio dei Dieci, Parti Comuni, Filza, Dicembre 1691.

5. For a broader discussion of Venetian attitudes towards irrigation and reclamation projects see Salvatore Ciriacono, *Acque e agricoltura Venezia: Olanda e la bonifica europea in età moderna* (Milan: Franco Angeli, 1994).

6. Pamela H. Smith, *The Body of the Artisan: Art and Experience in the Scientific Revolution* (Chicago: University of Chicago Press, 2004), p. 8; see also Pamela O.

Long, *Openness, Secrecy, Authorship: Technical Arts and the Culture of Knowledge from Antiquity to the Renaissance* (Baltimore: Johns Hopkins University Press, 2001), pp. 247–50.

7. Engineers would eventually have to defend their own brand of empirical knowledge against Newtonian natural philosophers. See Tal Golan, *Laws of Men and Laws of Nature: The History of Scientific Expert Testimony in England and America* (Cambridge, Mass.: Harvard University Press, 2004), pp. 5–51.

8. See Karl Appuhn, "Inventing Nature: Forests, Forestry and State Power in Renaissance Venice," *Journal of Modern History* 72 (2000): 861–90.

9. ASV, Savi ed esecutori alle acque (hereafter SEA), B. 72, c. 37 con all. includes the detailed cost estimate.

10. ASV, SEA, B. 72, c. 54r–v.

11. See for example, ASV, SEA, B. 72, c. 18, 28, and 32 for three rival proposals that were not given a field trial.

12. Gaetano Cozzi, "Storie e politica del dibatitto veneziano sulla laguna (Secc. XV–XVIII)," in *Conterminazione lagunare: Storia, ingegneria, politica, e diritto nella Laguna di Venezia* (Venice: Istituto Veneto di Scienze, Lettere ed Arti, 1992), p. 21.

13. Élisabeth Crouzet-Pavan, "Toward an Ecological Understanding of the Myth of Venice," in *Venice Reconsidered: The History and Civilization of an Italian City-State, 1297–1797,* ed. John Martin and Dennis Romano (Baltimore: Johns Hopkins University Press, 2000). pp. 39–65.

14. For a detailed discussion of the various dredging techniques employed in and around the lagoon see Roberto Berveglieri, *Le vie di Venezia: Canali lagunari e rii a Venezia: Inventori, brevetti, tecnologia e legislazione nei secoli XIII–XVIII* (Verona: Cierre, 1999), pp. 38–43.

15. For an account of the process of creating the hundreds of islands that make up the city and of the problems associated with building in such an environment, see Deborah Howard, *The Architectural History of Venice* (New York: Holmes and Meier, 1981); and Crouzet-Pavan, *"Sopra le acque salse."*

16. Giuseppe Pavanello, ed., *Marco Cornaro (1412–1464), scritture sulla laguna* (Venice: n.p., 1919). See also Crouzet-Pavan, *"Sopra le acque salse,"* p. 356; and Karl Appuhn, "Politics, Perception, and the Meaning of Landscape in Late Medieval Venice: Marco Cornaro's 1442 Inspection of Firewood Supplies," in *Inventing Medieval Landscapes: Senses of Place in Western Europe,* ed. John Howe and Michael Wolfe (Gainesville, Fla.: University Press of Florida, 2002), pp. 70–88. The most important later works on the lagoon include Cristoforo Sabbadino, *Discorsi sopra la laguna di Cristoforo Sabbadino,* vol. 2 of *Antichi scrittori d'idraulica veneta,* ed. Roberto Cessi (Venice: Ferrari, 1930); Nicolò Contarini, *Delle istorie veneziane,* in *Storici e politici veneti del Cinquecento e del Seicento,* ed. G. Benzoni and T. Zanato (Milan: Ricciardi, 1982), pp. 186–89; and Giovanni Correr, *Venezia e le sue lagune* (Venice: n.p., 1847).

17. Biblioteca Nazionale Marciana, It VII, 395 (8648).

18. Cozzi, "Storie e politica del dibatitto veneziano sulla laguna," p. 34.

19. See for example, Marino Sanuto, *I diarii di Marino Sanuto,* ed. R. Fulin et al., 58 vols. (Bologna: Forni Editore, 1879–1903), 12:89, for a reference to a major flood.

20. See, for example, ibid., 8:381.

21. See, for example, ibid., 7:588.

22. See for example the report in ASV, Senato Mar, Filza 549, c. nn., 23 March 1666.

23. A documentary history of the *savi ed esecutori alle acque* can be found in Giulio Rompiasio, *Metodo in pratica di sommario o sia compilazione delle leggi, terminazioni & ordini appartenenti agl'illustrissimi & eccelentissimi collegio e magistrato alle acque,* ed. Giovanni Caniato (Venice: Ministero per Ben i Culturali, 1988).

24. See, for example, Manfredo Tafuri, *Venice and the Renaissance* (Cambridge, Mass.: MIT Press, 1989); Cozzi, "Storie e politica del dibatitto veneziano sulla laguna"; and Ciriacono, *Acque e agricoltura.*

25. For a biography of Cornaro as well as critical editions of his most important treatises see Giuseppe Fiocco, *Alvise Cornaro: Il suo tempo e le sue opere* (Vicenza: Pozza, 1965).

26. Tafuri, *Venice and the Renaissance,* pp. 139–41.

27. Sabbadino, *Discorso sopra la laguna.*

28. Tafuri, *Venice and the Renaissance,* pp. 185–87.

29. For more on the *conterminazione* project, see the volume *Conterminazione lagunare: Storia, ingegneria, politica, e diritto nella Laguna di Venezia. Atti del convegno di studio nel bicentenario della conterminazione lagunare, Venezia 14–16 marzo 1991* (Venice: Istituto Veneto di Scienze, Lettere ed Arti, 1992).

30. For a case study of Venetian efforts to alter the inland watershed see Rafaello Vergani, *Brentella: Problemi d'acque nell'alta pianura trevigiana dei secoli XV e XVI* (Treviso: Canova, 2001).

31. Ciriacono, *Acque e agricoltura,* pp. 162–67.

32. Ibid., pp. 212–17; Berveglieri, *Le vie di Venezia;* and *Inventori stranieri a Venezia, 1474–1788* (Venice: Istituto Veneto di Scienze, Lettere ed Arti, 1995).

33. J. C. Eade, "The Accuracy of Vincenzo Coronelli's Celestial Globe," in *Isis* 68 (1977): 437–40. For more on Coronelli see *Dizionario biografico degli italiani,* vol. 29 (Rome, 1983), pp. 305–9; Comune di Venezia, *Vincenzo Coronelli cosmografo della serenissima: Nel terzo centenario dalla nascita* (Venice: n.p., 1950); James L. Fuchs, "Vincenzo Coronelli and the Organization of Knowledge: The Twilight of Seventeenth-Century Encyclopedism" (Ph.D. diss., University of Chicago, 1983); and Maria Gioia Tavoni, ed., *Un intellettuale europeo e il suo universo: Vincenzo Coronelli* (Bologna: Costa Editore, 1999).

34. Fuchs, "Vincenzo Coronelli," p. 66.

35. ASV, SEA, B. 72, c. 24.

36. ASV, SEA, B. 72, c. 37.

37. ASV, SEA, B. 72, c. 38.

38. ASV, Testamenti—Bronzini, B. 140, c. 201; and a later amendment can be found in ASV, Cancelleria Inferiore, Cedule, B. 70, c. 396.

39. ASV, SEA, B. 72, c. 41.

40. ASV, SEA, B. 72, c. 50.

41. ASV, SEA, B. 72, c. 54.

42. Ettore Scimeni, "Il Padre Coronelli idraulico," *Miscellanea Francescana* 51 (1951): 82–107.

6

Banking on Sacramento

Urban Development, Flood Control, and Political Legitimization, 1848–1862

Andrew C. Isenberg

In 1849, Elisha Crosby staked out his claim to a fortune in California. Crosby was not a prospector, however, but a city-builder. He and his two partners approached the cash-strapped Swiss-Mexican *empresario* Johann Sutter, who in 1838 had received a grant from the Mexican government of forty-eight thousand acres in the Sacramento Valley. They purchased from him eighteen hundred acres on the east bank of the Sacramento River at its juncture with the Feather River. There, Crosby and his partners laid out the lots for a town that they named "Vernon." They were not the only city-builders in the Central Valley. Farther south, Sutter's son John had begun to develop Sacramento City on what he assumed was part of his father's grant at the juncture of the Sacramento and American rivers. By the summer of 1850, John Sutter and his partners would discover that the elder Sutter's original grant had not included the lowlands where they had laid out Sacramento's lots. No one was aware of this oversight in 1849, however, as the developers of Sacramento, Vernon, and other towns scrambled to create a commercial center for the gold country.[1]

When James Marshall, one of Sutter's employees, had discovered gold on the south fork of the American River in January, 1848, most of the California interior was without a trace of urban settlement.[2] The Central Valley's closest approximation of an urban place was Sutter's seigneurial estate of New Helvetia, which had an Indian population of almost three thousand.[3] Following the discovery of gold, Sutter's Indian laborers abandoned the fiefdom as prospectors swept over his lands. By November, 1850, Isaac Owens, an itinerant Methodist minister, described Sutter's adobe fort as being in a "dilapidated state."[4]

The collapse of Sutter's settlement opened the opportunity for other sites to become the urban centers of the Gold Rush. Indeed, in mid-1849, Vernon "assumed quite a little importance as a trading point for the Feather River miner," according to Crosby. By autumn, Vernon had a population of over six hundred and seemed likely to become an important urban center for the mining region. Yet Vernon's great natural advantage—its position at the meeting point of two major rivers, the Feather and the Sacramento—also doomed its chances. "When the winter rains came in," according to Crosby, "that whole country was flooded, and one vast sea of water surrounded the little Elevation where the town was situated." The next year, a competing town-builder laid out the city of Marysville farther up the Feather River at its juncture with the Yuba. By the end of 1850, Marysville and Sacramento had emerged as the primary urban centers for the mines to the east. So complete was the triumph of Marysville and Sacramento that their residents cannibalized Vernon's abandoned buildings. Within four years, Vernon had vanished.[5]

Like the ill-fated Vernon, the cities that eventually emerged as the leading commercial centers of the Central Valley—Sacramento, Marysville, and Stockton—hardly existed as settlements as late as 1848. Like Crosby and his partners, the founders of Sacramento, Marysville, and Stockton imagined that their cities would become centers of commerce for the gold-mining territory to the east. The imperative of commerce dictated their selection of town sites: like Crosby, they chose places at the juncture of major rivers: Sacramento at the meeting of the American and Sacramento rivers; Marysville at the juncture of the Feather and Yuba rivers; and Stockton near the point where the Calaveras River joins the San Joaquin River. At these places, merchants and miners disembarked from their watercraft and set out overland for the gold country.[6]

To contemporaries, nature, in the Sacramento–San Joaquin river system, seemed to provide the routes to commercial wealth. "Looking at a map of California," J. D. Borthwick observed in 1857, "the Sacramento river running parallel with the mines, the San Joaquin joining it from the southward and eastward, and the Feather river continuing a northward course from the Sacramento—all of them being navigable—present the natural means of communication between San Francisco and the 'mines.'" In accordance with this geocommercial logic, Sacramento, Marysville, and Stockton "sprang up," each as a "depôt" for the mines in its vicinity, "with roads radiating from it across the plains to the various settlements in the mountains."[7]

Yet the emergence of the Central Valley cities as economic nodes for the gold country was neither an automatic nor a natural phenomenon, however much the long-standing tradition of scholarship in urban studies that views cities as evolving "organisms" might make it seem.[8] The Central Valley cities had been founded as speculative enterprises, and for the rest of the nineteenth century their governments and their residents alike continued to promote commerce actively in order to expand. In an 1854 editorial, the Whig journal the *Marysville Herald* explained the competitive venture of urban development. Marysville, the editors wrote, was the third largest city in the state, and "will soon be rivaled only by San Francisco. But how to promote its growth—to place its advancement beyond the possibility of a doubt? Why, simply, to increase our trade."[9] Cities such as Marysville and Sacramento were rather more like joint-stock companies than organisms. Merchants and speculators in real estate were the investors in these companies; municipal governments, made up largely of the most prominent land speculators and merchants, acted as boards of directors.[10]

For the cities to emerge as commercial centers of the gold country, municipal governments had to construct means of transportation both to the coast and to the Sierra foothills. For example, while the rivers that joined at Marysville were an important natural advantage for the city, the municipal government was determined to improve the commercial possibilities of the streams. Thus, the Marysville City Charter provided the municipal government with the power to "grade the banks of the Yuba and Feather Rivers, so as to facilitate the discharge of merchandize from steamers, vessels, and boats."[11] Likewise, in 1854, Marysville residents voted overwhelmingly to build a railroad to Benicia and a plank road to Nevada City.[12]

Sacramento's city government had even grander ambitions. In 1853, the city council sought to issue bonds to finance the construction of a railroad to the interior.[13] In 1855, the city granted a right of way to the Sacramento Valley Railroad Company. By 1856, the company had laid twenty-two miles of track along the American River as far as Folsom. The company hoped its line would become the western leg of a transcontinental railroad.[14] In short, the economic growth of Sacramento Valley cities was not an inexorable process, but the result of deliberate choices by the cities' leaders.

Yet the proximity of the rivers that made this growth possible was a curse as well as a blessing: just as Vernon flooded in the winter of 1849–50, Sacramento, Marysville, and Stockton flooded repeatedly in the nineteenth century. (Indeed, Marysville residents eventually rued the day that they had graded the riverbank.) The urbanization of nineteenth-century California was thus not a simple story of cities rising from the wilderness, as nineteenth-century boosters (and historians) imagined it to be. Rather, the rise of urban centers in the decades after the discovery of gold was a complex and often contradictory phenomenon: positioned to profit from the exploitation of nature, cities found themselves in the path of natural catastrophe. Commerce in natural resources built the Central Valley cities, but the ecology of commerce brought flood. City governments thus faced an ecological dilemma: to mitigate the threat to their urban environment by levying taxes and creating levees, they had to restrain the commerce that was the source of prosperity. Yet municipal public works projects, despite their expense, imparted significant political benefits to city governments: such projects conferred political legitimacy on governments that had been initially conceived as little more than real estate development companies.

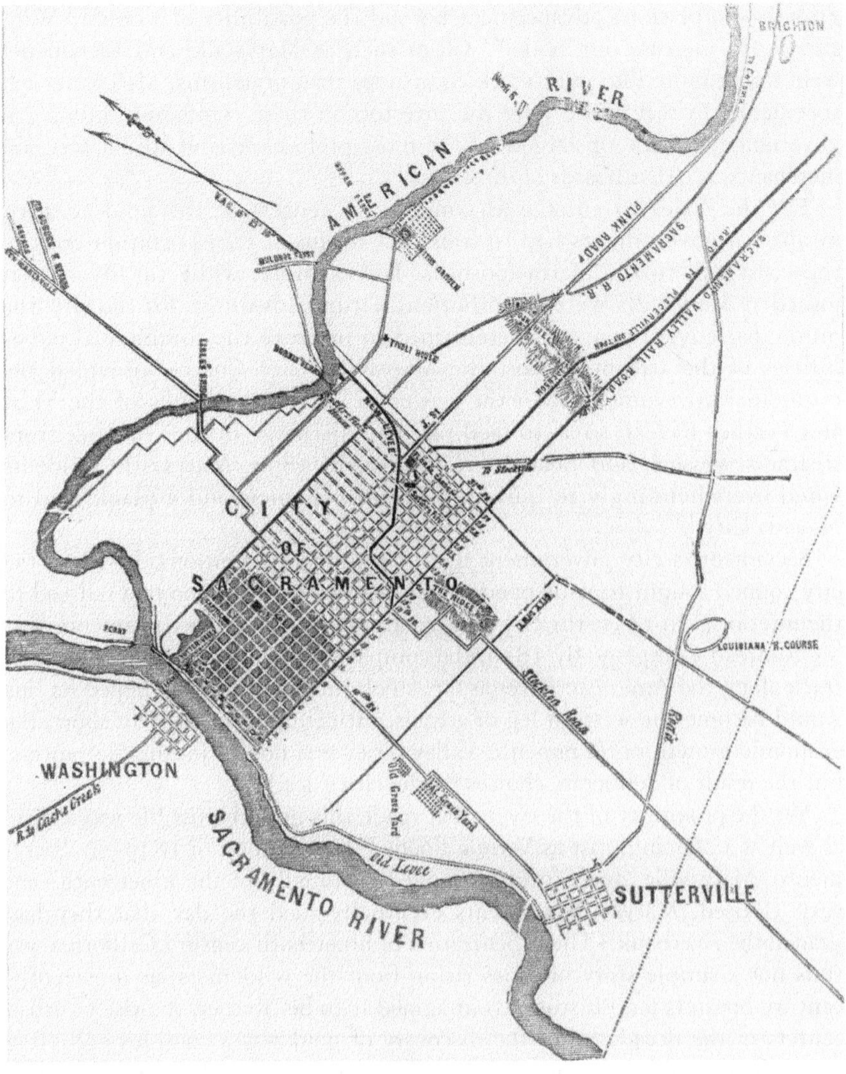

Map 1. Sacramento and vicinity, c. 1855. Courtesy Sacramento Archives and Museum Collection Center.

If ever a city's birth was illegitimate, then it was the founding of Sacramento. In December 1848, while Johann Sutter was hiding from his creditors, his son John, acting in his place, entered into an agreement with Peter Burnett, later the governor of California, to develop Sacramento City. The elder Sutter would not have approved of the scheme, if for no other reason than that he had already staked his urban development plans on Sutterville, the town he had founded in 1844 downstream from the juncture of the American and Sacramento rivers. In January, 1849, Burnett and the younger Sutter lured the principal Sutterville merchants, Sam Brannan, Barton Lee, and Albert Priest, to Sacramento by offering them each five hundred city lots to move their operations to Sacramento. Leaving nothing to chance, Brannan and other Sacramento merchants, now effectively partners in the city's development scheme, descended on the one large commercial establishment remaining in Sutterville and destroyed its stock of goods.[15]

Merchant-speculators dominated the Sacramento city government. Brannan and Lee had served on the committee to draft laws for the provisional government of California; both served on the board of commissioners to draft laws for Sacramento. Other members of the board included the merchants William Petit and William Carpenter; John Fowler, a sometime partner of Brannan who had a near-monopoly on freighting between Sacramento and the mines; and John McDougal, a real estate investor in Sacramento and later a governor of California. The first city government, elected in April 1850, included Lee as city treasurer; Hardin Bigelow, a merchant and real estate speculator, as mayor; and as members of the city council the merchant-speculators Demas Strong and James Hardenburgh. In short, a list of the most prominent businessmen in Sacramento in 1849 and 1850 was virtually indistinguishable from the roster of the city government.[16]

By October 1849, Sacramento had a population of over two thousand. The rapid growth of the city outpaced construction supplies: of the nearly 350 buildings in the fall of 1849, 85 percent were hastily assembled of wooden frames with canvas walls and roofs. Lumber was too expensive in 1849 for all but the most extravagant builders to consider a construction entirely of wood.[17] Merchants scrambled to acquire the best commercial spaces. Isaac Perkins, who migrated from Massachusetts to Sacramento, arriving in April, 1850, quickly concluded that the success of his dry goods business depended on "getting a good location. It is here just as it is everywhere else some parts of the city you could not sell enough to pay your expenses wilst in others you can sell all the goods you can get."[18] In the scramble for space, some speculators made fortunes in the commerce in city lots. Some lots sold for as much as $8,000 in 1849. When Sacramento assessed property taxes for the first time in 1850, Brannan's property in the city was valued at over $26,000, and Lee's at over $22,000.[19]

Gradually, Sacramento began to assume a more citified appearance, replacing canvas buildings with wooden structures. To supply Sacramento with lumber, loggers cut immense numbers of trees on the American, Sacramento, and Feather rivers. On the American River alone, loggers cut a million board feet of lumber in 1852 and four million board feet in 1853.[20] By May 1850, the price of lumber, which had stood as high as $1.50 per foot in Sacramento a year earlier, had fallen to three cents per foot. "Lumber is extremely plenty and there is great quantity in this market," wrote one observer in Sacramento.[21] Loggers' industriousness may have lowered the price of lumber in Sacramento, but it contributed to the destruction of the dense forests of the Central Valley riverbanks above Sacramento.[22] Below Sacramento, increasing steamboat travel deforested the riverbanks, as steamboats consumed wood for fuel and cut trees from the riverbanks to prevent snags.[23]

The consumption of the riverine forests exacerbated the lowlands' inherent tendency to flood. Deforestation removed trees whose dense roots had stabilized the natural levees flanking the rivers, and loggers' practice of floating their timber downstream to urban markers furthered erosion. According to an 1854 report, when loggers pushed the logs they had cut into the flood-swollen rivers in the spring, the logs, "thunder down the rapids, sometimes end over end, until they bring up on some rocky point or sand bar."[24] Such logging debris jams forced currents around obstructions in the river, scouring banks and levees in the process. Altogether, logging left the rivers in such a condition that floodwaters were more likely to transcend the streambed.[25]

Floods occur regularly in the dynamic environment of the Sacramento River and its thirteen largest tributaries, which together drain a watershed area of over 58,000 square miles. The volume of water in the rivers that flow from the Sierra is unpredictable. Fifty percent of the flow is snowmelt from the upper Sierra, and the amount of snowfall in the mountains and the rate at which it melts—factors that vary considerably from year to year—largely determine the amount and the timing of spring floods. At Soda Springs, at an elevation of 6,900 feet, an average of eighty inches of snow usually accumulates between November and the end of March. Much of the upper Sierra usually accumulates sixty inches of snow each winter. The amount of moisture in winter storms can increase greatly during El Niño years, when pulses of warm water extend from the western to the eastern Pacific and wet winter storms produce heavy snowpacks in the Sierra. In such years, Soda Springs amasses an average of 160 inches of snow. If snowpacks melt gradually, their impact on streams dissipates, but if heavy snowfalls are followed by warm, midwinter rains in the upper Sierra, the snowpack melts rapidly.[26]

If the volume of water in the rivers that flow from the Sierra is unpredictable, so too is the course those rivers follow when they reach the floor of the Central Valley. Because rivers cross a variety of geological formations, their rate of flow is uneven. Narrow streams confined by rocky canyon walls have rapid currents; the currents of broader streams are slow. Currents change speed as they flow across riffles, or high points, in the streambed. Water accumulates in deep pools at bends in a river, where it increases in pressure and, accordingly, downstream speed. Riffles and pools create the meandering shape of the Central Valley rivers. Such meanders are not static: especially during spring floods, high waters create cutoffs between meanders, leaving the old streambeds as oxbows or sloughs.[27]

Snowmelt brought flood to Sacramento in January 1850, just as it had to Elisha Crosby's settlement of Vernon. The *Alta California* reported a "vast lake of waters" from Sacramento to Sutter's Fort, submerging all but the tops of trees for miles. The flood made a mockery of Sacramento's commercial aspirations: "lumber, bales and cases of goods, boxes and barrels, tents and small houses were floating in every direction." The city's inhabitants clustered on a bluff above the town until the water receded some two weeks later. In its wake, the flood left "many gullies in which was deposited all the filth of the surrounding neighborhood."[28]

The flood did more than expose the folly of Sacramento's location in the low-lying flood plain at the juncture of two major rivers. The flood also revealed the limits of Johann Sutter's Mexican land grant which was the legal basis for the development of Sacramento—and, thus, for the wealth that speculation in city lots had produced. The Mexican government had never formally deeded the land to Sutter; moreover, the grant specifically excluded the riverine land on which Sacramento City stood. Sutter, intending to found an upland agricultural estate, had been content to exclude "overflowed" land from his grant. By late 1849, a number of settlers in Sacramento had disdained the purchase of lots and merely "squatted" on the land without title. Squatters settled in particular on the natural levee along the Sacramento River, and challenged the legitimacy of Sutter's grant. John Plumbe, one of the leaders of the squatters, who formed themselves into a "Settlers Association," discovered the limited extent of Sutter's property in the spring of 1850, when he secured a copy of the grant.[29] In the absence of a clear title, squatters argued that the land was part of the public domain. They appealed to American custom and the legal tradition of preemption that generally accorded title to those who occupied and improved public land.

Speculators, who styled themselves the "Law and Order Party," used the power of the city government they controlled to evict the squatters. The city removed most squatters from the levee in December, 1849—a few weeks before floodwaters would have removed them anyway. Shortly after the eviction, the Law and Order Party called a public meeting intending to endorse the legality of the Sutter grant; they quickly discovered that the majority of attenders at the meeting sympathized with the squatters. By this time the squatters and their sympathizers held the speculators' city government in open contempt. "The squatters," wrote the overland migrant Israel Lord, who arrived in the city in December 1849, "had as much right to the land where Sacramento City stands as anybody (certainly more than the swindling minions of Sutter)."[30] The Settlers Association complained of "threats of violence" and "brute force" by the city government. They derided the legitimacy of the "so-called legislature of California" which had certified Sacramento City's charter, and the city's "legislative regulations, by them called *laws*."[31]

Facing a hostile majority in the city, the Sacramento speculators prosecuted a suit against the squatters in the county court; in August 1850, the court decided against the squatters, prompting a riot in the city. During a day of violence on 14 August, a dozen squatters and several city officials, including the sheriff and the city assessor, were killed. Burnett, by then governor of California, ordered the state militia to restore order. The city declared martial law; within days the rioting squatters had been subdued, and the city had established its authority—if not, in the eyes of many observers, its legitimacy.[32]

The squatters' riot was the formative political event in Sacramento's first decade; it cast a shadow over the city into the 1860s as successive city administrations struggled to establish their legitimacy. Yet in the immediate aftermath of the riot, the municipal government did little to show that it was anything more than the head office of a land development company. In the fall of 1850, the city government was forced to confront an epidemic of cholera. By that time, Sacramento had already become a city with more than its share of illness. Many migrants by land and sea to California arrived in Sacramento exhausted and suffering from a variety of illnesses; moreover those who fell ill in the gold country sought medical care in Sacramento.[33] As the sick congregated in the city, according to the Sacramento physician John Morse, "Sacramento became a perfect lazar house of disease, suffering, and death months before anything like an effective city government was organized."[34] The sick congregated in small private hospitals constructed—usually of canvas—by physicians themselves.[35]

Newcomers to Sacramento, whether healthy or ill, arrived in a crowded, dirty city. By the early summer of 1850, Sacramento's population had inflated to seven thousand. Most Sacramento residents simply dumped refuse in city streets; the city, unwilling to commit public resources to efforts that had no direct economic benefits, made no effort to clear the streets of waste.[36] On 20 October 1850, Israel Lord wrote in his journal that "This evening the streets are as filthy as ever, and the heated city is a living, moving, tailing mass of men and animals, crawling like maggots in the filth, and breathing an atmosphere filled with poison and dust. The smoke and dust form a dense cloud, which involves everything in obscurity."[37] In Sacramento's first year, the standards of public health slipped thus to a dangerously low level.

In October, an epidemic of cholera struck the city. In 1849, trade and migration had brought the disease to the North American West. The cholera bacterium, *Vibrio comma,* which survived in watering holes along the overland trail, accompanied emigrants to California: two thousand overland emigrants died of cholera in the late 1840s and 1850s.[38] Alas for Sacramento in 1850, cholera is a disease that thrives in conditions of urban filth. The bacterium can be transmitted from one host to another through unwashed hands or raw sewage. When raw sewage containing the bacterium finds its way into the public water supply, cholera spreads rapidly.[39] The disease strikes without warning: its symptoms are severe abdominal pain, vomiting, and diarrhea. In the course of a single day, it can be fatal to an otherwise healthy person. Perkins wrote on 27 October that "Some have been taken who were to all appearances in Good Health & have died in a few hours."[40] On October 23, for instance, Lord noted in his journal, "A man walking down J street last evening, dropped suddenly, and lived only long enough to be carried into the nearest door."[41]

The first death from cholera occurred on 20 October. The number of cases rapidly multiplied over the next few weeks, radiating into the city from the commercial riverside district: seven deaths by 22 October; between fifteen and twenty more by 24 October; and a further thirty to forty by 26 October. Lord estimated that during the twenty days that the disease raged through Sacramento, eight hundred people died. The *Alta California* reported that at the height of the epidemic sixty people died every day. Public health measures proved to be worse than ineffective. A city ordinance passed on 21 October ordered residents to burn their garbage or face a five-hundred-dollar fine. Lord wrote that "the filth is burned in the middle of the streets—old shoes and boots and clothes by the ton, and cart loads of bones, and raw hides, and putrid meat, and spoiled bacon—so that the end of the matter is worse than the beginning." By the end of the month, half of the population of Sacramento had either succumbed to the disease or fled the city. By the end of the first week of November, by the reckoning of both Lord and Morse, 80 percent had either died or fled. The exodus included several members of the Sacramento city council. "There are a thousand things which call loudly for supervision, but in vain," complained the San Francisco *Alta California* on 3 November. "No means have been taken to disinfect the atmosphere (at least by the city), no precautions against the accumulation of filth."[42]

By the end of 1850, the municipal government of Sacramento faced a crisis of legitimacy. It had shot its way into power in August and displayed apathy and cravenness before and during the cholera epidemic of October and November. For one project, however, the city government enjoyed public support: its efforts to build a levee to protect the city from flood. Such efforts were initially the work of business leaders seeking to protect their investments. In late January 1850, in the wake of the flood of 1849–50, Barton Lee called a meeting to discuss a levee. A fellow merchant and speculator, Hardin Bigelow, was appointed to head the levee committee. The city council, always wary of public expenses, delayed action on Bigelow's recommendations, however, so when ten inches of rain fell in March 1850, Bigelow hired a workforce at his own expense and supervised the construction of a makeshift levee. The city was not inundated, and Bigelow was promptly acclaimed as a civic hero; when the city held its first municipal elections on 1 April, he was elected mayor.[43] He immediately called for a referendum on the question of raising $250,000 in taxes to construct a levee; the measure passed in late April by a vote of 543 to 15.[44]

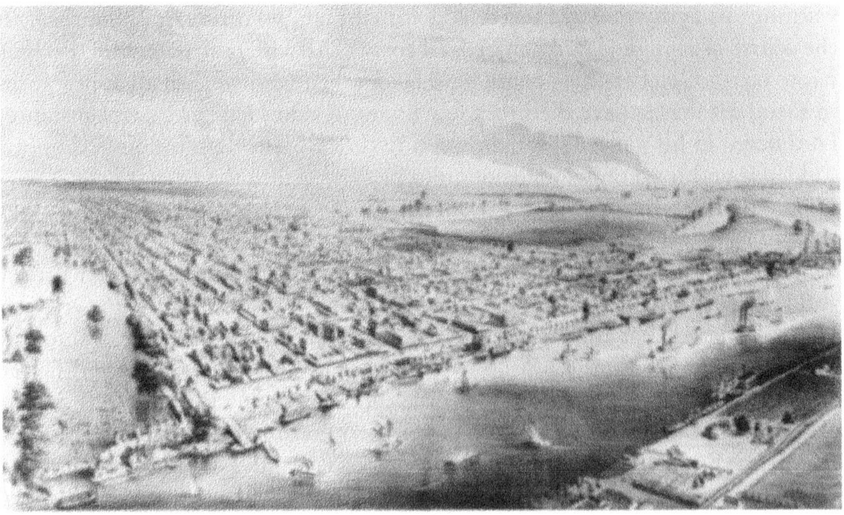

Figure 1. Sacramento and its rivers, c. 1857. Courtesy Sacramento Archives and Museum Collection Center.

Bigelow's promising political career was cut short by Sacramento's chaos, however: he was shot by squatters during the August riots, and while recovering from his wounds, he died of cholera in November. Bigelow's astute use of flood control to build political popularity was taken up by James Hardenburgh, who became chair of the city's levee committee in September. Hardenburgh supervised the construction of a levee nine miles in length. A section of the levee three feet high, six feet broad at the crest, and twelve feet wide at the base ran along the American River; along the Sacramento River the embankment rose to six feet high, fourteen feet broad at its crest, and thirty feet wide at its base. The construction, completed at the end of 1850, cost $175,000 at a time when the city's expenses for all other purposes totaled only $100,000.[45] In contrast to its unenthusiastic response to Bigelow's request for funds in March 1850, the city council was eager to take on the expense of the levee as a sign of both its indispensability and its public-spiritedness.

Construction necessitated condemning some private property along the waterfront.[46] The transformation of this area, the center of the squatters' movement, to city property was the final triumph of the city over the Settlers Association. As public property, the levee was an embodiment of the municipal government. More than protection from flood, it was a cordon along the city's boundary to solidify the city government's tenuous claim to authority; it was a bulwark against challenges from within and without.[47]

Whatever the levee's symbolic value, its efficacy as protection against flooding was dubious. The flood of January 1850 had merely presaged a more extensive flood in the spring of 1852, when Sacramento, Marysville, and Stockton were inundated. In Marysville, the floodwaters overflowed the city's business district.[48] The floodwaters continued on to Sacramento: on 7 March, the level of the American River as it passed Sacramento rose at a rate of one foot per hour, and the water breached the city levee on the Sacramento River at I Street. The waters of the American also poured into a slough outside of the city. By 11 March, the water of the slough was three feet higher than the city, and water poured steadily from it into Sacramento. The city's residents hastily built a levee along J Street to hold back the waters, but their construction collapsed overnight.[49]

The damage to property and business notwithstanding, the floods of the early 1850s were mere trickles compared to the flood of the winter and spring of 1861–62, when unusually heavy snowmelts encountered streambeds raised by hydraulic mining debris. Unaware of this alignment of forces, Sacramento residents welcomed the commercial potential of the first rains of the season in November 1861. The rain, the *Sacramento Daily Union* opined, would "start grain and grass, and enable farmers to commence plowing on lowland. This will give life and activity to business operations in agricultural districts." Reports of rain in Grass Valley caused the *Daily Union* to welcome the "plentiful supply of the element so essential to the prosperity of the miner." The newspaper was still joking about rising waters later in the month, noting that at a slaughterhouse south of Sacramento on the road to Stockton, 250 rats had been drowned.[50]

Sacramento residents had reason to feel secure that the fate of the rats was not a portent. Nine years had passed since the last flood, "a time so long that many of our citizens had concluded that the city was safe from damage by water," wrote the *Daily Union.* Yet the city government had also taken constructive steps to protect Sacramento. Since the floods of 1852, the city government, at considerable expense, had extended the 1850 structure to ring the city with a levee. The two principal parts of the levee were on the banks of the Sacramento and American rivers: alongside the Sacramento it ran south from the mouth of the American as far as Sutterville, and alongside the American it extended from the juncture with the Sacramento eastward for three miles. In addition, a levee ran eastward along R Street from the Sacramento River levee as far as Sixteenth Street, turned to the northeast and continued to the city limits at Thirty-first Street, and then ran north along Thirty-first Street until it joined the American River levee. For added security, the city government spent eight thousand dollars in 1860 to build a wing-dam that jutted into the American River to direct the current away from the city levee and toward the opposite bank.[51]

While the city government raised the levee around Sacramento, other California enterprises were raising the beds of the Sacramento and American rivers. As early as 1852, engineers in the gold country had begun to use pressurized water from a reservoir to flush gold-bearing gravel through a sluice. The technique substantially lowered labor costs. but significant amounts of debris found their way into the rivers that drained westward from the foothills of the Sierra Nevada. By the end of the 1850s, such hydraulic mining operations on the Feather, Bear, Yuba, and American rivers—all of which drained into the Sacramento—were extensive.[52] A farmer who had settled on the Yuba in 1851 claimed that at certain points along the river, tailings had covered twenty-foot tall telegraph poles so fully that only the top four to six feet remained above the surface.[53] While larger pieces of debris accumulated in the higher ravines, the current carried still more waste in the form of smaller, lighter amounts of sand and soil farther downstream.[54] The lighter debris filled river channels, transforming the swift, clear rivers flowing from the Sierra into slow, murky, broad effluents. James H. Keyes, who settled on a farm along the Bear in 1856 described it at that time as "a clear, running stream, with well-defined banks." After 1860, however, the bed began to fill. The sediment "has entirely obliterated the channel, running over the bottomlands in every direction." Likewise, the channel of the Yuba was filled so completely with hydraulic mining sediment that the stream ran a mile away from its original course.[55]

The raised riverbeds of the Yuba, Bear, Feather, and Sacramento caused spring freshets to inundate riverine farmlands with a watery mixture of sand and gravel that farmers dubbed "slickens."[56] On the Yuba River, slickens covered one farmer's bottomlands with over eight feet of sediment. In order to confine the waters of the spring freshets, farmers raised the levees along the rivers, and as new deposits of sediment accreted on the riverbeds, they raised the levees further. Within two decades of the onset of hydraulic mining, stretches of the Bear River's bed were actually higher than the surrounding countryside. Only the walls of the levees kept the waters of the river from overflowing.[57]

Against such transformed rivers, the Sacramento City levee was not impregnable. In March 1861, spring freshets severely damaged the wing-dam, and by the fall the damage had yet to be repaired.[58] Yet Sacramento remained safely barricaded by its levee while towns upriver were overwhelmed by the floodwaters of late 1861 and early 1862. In Auburn on 8 December, floodwaters swept away a number of houses. The flood reached Marysville at eleven o'clock in the evening of 9 December. By the early morning of 10 December, floodwaters in Marysville were so high that a steamboat made its way through the city streets rescuing citizens trapped on roofs or in the upper stories of buildings. An observer reported that the agricultural land south of Marysville was a "waste of muddy water, on which are floating houses, fences, lumber, hay, straw, and the dead and living bodies of hogs, cattle, and horses." Indeed, livestock was "constantly passing down stream, some alive and struggling, and bellowing and squealing for life."[59]

On the morning of 9 December, the floodwaters breached Sacramento's levees, not, as was feared, in the northwest corner of the city, below the damaged wing-dam, where the swollen American River flowed into the equally swollen Sacramento, but in the southeast corner of the city. There, a railroad line designed to bring commercial traffic into the city accidentally allowed floodwaters into Sacramento. The American River had breached the levee upriver of Sacramento, and proceeded to pour into a dry slough on the west of the city. The rising waters abutted against an embankment constructed a few years earlier by the Sacramento Valley Railroad Company, which ran across the slough and entered the city at the corner of R and Sixteenth Streets, the southeast corner of the city levee. The city ordinance granting the railroad its right of way had stipulated that the company was to build a bridge across the slough, allowing water to pass beneath it. The company had constructed a bridge in 1855, but in the two years before the flood the bridge had fallen into disrepair. To shore up the structure, the company had transformed the bridge into an embankment by filling in its spans with earth. By the time of the flood of December 1861, the embankment was higher than the levee on the southeast side of the city. Floodwater flowing into the slough from the American River abutted against the embankment and rose until it overtopped the levee and poured into the city.[60] In both Sacramento and Marysville, where the flood had poured into the city at a point where the levee had been graded to facilitate steamboat traffic, the flood followed the gates of commerce into the cities.

After entering Sacramento at the railroad embankment at six o'clock in the morning, the floodwaters gushed through the southern part of the city, submerging one-story houses to their rooftops. By nine o'clock, the city south of J Street was under water. The flood exposed the weakness of the city's vaunted system of levees: once the river breached or overtopped any part of the twelve miles of levees encircling the city, the embankments, rather than keeping floodwaters out, kept them in. To drain water from the southern part of the city, residents opened breaches in the levee to let water out. The waters flowed in such force through the openings that they carried a number of houses through them.[61]

By mid-December, it appeared that the crisis had passed. Water had largely, although not entirely, receded from the southern part of the city. North of L Street, the city had remained dry. Teams of workers set about to repair the damaged levee in early January, 1862, and a barge loaded with 100,000 feet of lumber arrived to rebuild the Sacramento Valley Railroad at R Street. Sacramento's boosters remained optimistic in the face of flood. "When the weather clears up," the *Daily Union* confidently predicted on 10 January, "the streets and bridges leading to and from the city will be repaired and built, and Sacramento will resume her trade and activity as if nothing unusual had happened."[62]

That very evening, however, the city was flooded again. The flood originated in this instance from the Sacramento rather than the American River; the level of the Sacramento was half a foot higher on 10 January than it had been on 9 December. Unlike the deluge of 9 December, the flood of 10 January began slowly, as water in the still submerged southern parts of the city began rising and seeping northward. It then rose rapidly, drowning four city residents and five inhabitants of a ranch outside the city. By the evening, the water within the city had reached the level of the Front Street levee and was lapping over it at places. Workers feverishly shored up the American River levee to prevent that from giving way as well. On 21 January, the *Daily Union,* ever confident, reported that as a result of these labors, "the levee was considered by good judges to be entirely safe." Two days later the repaired levee collapsed, and a "strong current" of water began flowing through the eastern part of the city, from the break on the American River south to openings in the R Street levee.[63] The American River had, in effect, transformed the eastern side of Sacramento into a cutoff.

In the aftermath of the 1861–62 flood, the Sacramento municipal government raised the city's levees still higher. By 1863, they were four feet higher than the flood stage of 1862. When the American River threatened to overwhelm the levee in 1867, the city added five more feet. The next year, the city government borrowed a tactic from the river itself. If in 1862 the river had used city streets as a cutoff, the city council in 1868 determined to create a cutoff that would reroute the American River's current away from Sacramento. The city paid for the digging of a canal from the point where the Central Pacific Railroad crossed the American River upstream from the city to a point one mile north of the American's juncture with the Sacramento, thereby directing most of the flow of the American River away from the city.[64]

Yet in February 1878, the city flooded again. Hydraulic mining debris was a significant contributor to the 1878 flood: sediment had continued to raise the bed of the American River, diminishing the effectiveness of Sacramento's towering levee. The effectiveness of the levee was also diminished by humbler means: while the levee was an artificial construction, the earthen structure was rapidly incorporated into the natural environment. Significant numbers of burrowing rodents made their homes in the levee by 1878, and its collapse in February of that year occurred in part because gophers had weakened it considerably. The break in the levee occurred south of the city, and the waters flooded the lowlands and then seeped into Sacramento as far north as N Street and as far east as Sixth Street.[65]

The founders of Sacramento had placed their settlement at the juncture of the Sacramento and American rivers because of the natural advantages that the streams offered. Within a few years, however, proximity to the rivers had become a distinct disadvantage. Once confident that they would profit from their location, the city's residents, like those of other cities in the valley, came to believe that they would profit despite it. Yet floods destroyed Vernon and handicapped Marysville's commercial prospects; the latter city's population declined significantly after the flood of 1852. Sacramento survived only by constructing levees and canals to protect it from the unpredictable American River. Sacramento embarked upon its flood control projects not because it was the wealthiest of the Central Valley cities, nor because it had the brightest prospects, but ironically because its government, lacking even a shadow of legitimacy, intuited that a flood control project might boost public support. Sacramento speculators who had touted the natural advantages of the city's location in 1850 trumpeted the artificial advantages of the city's levees in the 1860s. Sacramento was founded as a city that relied on nature for its commercial prospects; in little over a decade, it became a city that relied on artificial constructions to protect it from nature. The city levee failed to protect the city during the flood of 1861–62, but it was nonetheless a legitimization of the municipal government, and in a broader sense a validation of the artificial hydrology that hydraulic mining had created in California.

NOTES

1. Elisha Oscar Crosby Memoirs, Huntington Library, San Marino, California (hereafter HUN). For the founding of Sacramento, see J. S. Holliday, *Rush for Riches: Gold Fever and the Making of California* (Berkeley: University of California Press, 1999), p. 77.

2. *Stockton City Directory and Emigrant's Guide to the Southern Mines* (Stockton: San Joaquin Republican, 1852), p. 25.

3. *Sacramento Illustrated* (Sacramento: Barker and Baker, 1855), p. 15. For Indian labor at Sutter's fort, see Albert L. Hurtado, *Indian Survival on the California Frontier* (New Haven, Conn.: Yale University Press, 1988), pp. 55–71.

4. Isaac Owens Diary, 10 November 1850, HUN.

5. Elisha Oscar Crosby Memoirs.

6. Geographers call such places "breaks in transport": such places have become the sites of major North American cities. See Richard C. Wade, *The Urban Frontier: The Rise of Western Cities, 1780–1830* (Cambridge, Mass.: Harvard University Press, 1959); William Cronon, *Nature's Metropolis: Chicago and the Great West* (New York: Norton, 1991); Ari Kelman, *A River and Its City: The Nature of Landscape in New Orleans* (Berkeley: University of California Press, 2003).

7. J. D. Borthwick, *Three Years in California* (Oakland, Calif.: Biobooks, 1948), p. 80. Sacramento, Marysville, and Stockton created what urban historians and geographers call "nodal regions": territories that funneled their natural resources through an urban center. Taken together, the areas around the three cities also constituted a so-called "uniform region," dominated by the production of a primary commodity, gold. See Carl Abbott, "Frontiers and Sections: Cities and Regions in American

Growth," *American Quarterly* 37 (1985): 395–96. For nodal regions in the American West, see Donald W. Meinig, *Imperial Texas: An Interpretive Essay in Cultural Geography* (Austin: University of Texas Press, 1969); Cronon, *Nature's Metropolis.*

8. For the idea of cities as organisms, see Robert E. Park, "The City: Suggestions for the Investigation of Human Behavior in the City Environment," *American Journal of Sociology* 20 (March 1915): 577–612; Louis Wirth, "Human Ecology," *American Journal of Sociology* 50 (May 1945): 483–88; Spenser W. Havelick, *The Urban Organism* (New York: Macmillan, 1974); Peter G. Goheen, "Industrialization and the Growth of Cities in Nineteenth-Century America," *American Studies* 14 (1974): 49–65. For an analysis of the history of this idea, see Graeme Davison, "The City as a Natural System: Theories of Urban Society in Nineteenth-Century Britain,' in *The Pursuit of Urban History,* ed. Derek Fraser and Anthony Sutcliffe (London: Arnold, 1983).

9. *Marysville Herald,* 24 March 1854.

10. Such enterprises were common in the American West. See J. Christopher Schnell and Katherine Clinton, "The New West: Themes in Nineteenth-Century Urban Promotion, 1815–1880," *Missouri Historical Society Bulletin* 30 (1974): 75–88; Gilbert Stelter, "The City and Westward Expansion: A Western Case Study," *Western Historical Quarterly* 4 (1973): 187–202.

11. *Hale & Emery's Marysville City Directory* (Marysville: Marysville Herald, 1853), p. 13.

12. The railroad was to cost $800,000; the plank road $350,000. Benicia later voted to subscribe $250,000 to the cost of the railroad. *Marysville Herald,* 28 February, 6 and 10 March 1854.

13. City Council Minutes, 29 January 1853, City of Sacramento Public Archives.

14. The Sacramento Valley Railroad Company's line was superseded by the Central Pacific Railroad, which reached Sacramento by an alternate route. By 1870, the Central Pacific had driven the Sacramento Valley Railroad Company into a steep decline in business. See Francis A. Bishop to Placerville and Sacramento Valley Railroad Company, 19 February 1870, Bishop Letterbook, Francis Augustus Bishop Papers, HUN.

15. *Sacramento Illustrated,* pp. 24–26; Mark A. Eifler, *Gold Rush Capitalists: Greed and Growth in Sacramento* (Albuquerque: University of New Mexico Press, 2002), p. 52.

16. *Sacramento Illustrated,* pp. 38–39; Eifler, *Gold Rush Capitalists,* p. 64.

17. Thomas H. Thompson and Albert Augustus West, *History of Sacramento County, California* (Oakland: Thompson & West, 1880), p. 146.

18. Isaac Perkins to Daniel Perkins, 28 April 1850, Isaac Perkins Correspondence, California State Library, Sacramento.

19. *Sacramento Illustrated,* pp. 38–39; Eifler, *Gold Rush Capitalists,* p. 64.

20. "Lumbermen Cutting Saw-Logs on the American," *Sacramento Daily Union,* 17 November 1854.

21. Samuel Nichols to Sarah Ann Nichols, 8 May 1850, Samuel Nichols Collection, HUN.

22. Kenneth Thompson, "Riparian Forests of the Sacramento Valley, California," *Annals of the Association of American Geographers* 51 (September 1961): 294–315.

23. For deforestation by steamboats, see Kelman, *A River and Its City,* p. 67.

24. "Lumbermen Cutting Saw-Logs on the American."

25. Jeffrey F. Mount, *California Rivers and Streams: The Conflict between Fluvial Process and Land Use* (Berkeley: University of California Press, 1995), pp. 56–57, 236.

26. Mount, *California Rivers and Streams,* pp. 83–100, 145–60; Thompson, "Riparian Forests of the Sacramento Valley," p. 300.

27. Mount, *California Rivers and Streams,* pp. 52–82.

28. "Flood at Sacramento City," *Alta California,* 14 January 1850; "Sacramento and Placer Intelligence," Ibid., 6 February 1850.

29. John Plumbe, *The Settlers and Land Speculators of Sacramento* (1851), p. 13. See also *Sacramento Illustrated,* p. 42.

30. Israel Lord quoted in Peter Blodgett, *Land of Golden Dreams: California in the Gold Rush Decade, 1848–1858* (San Marino, Calif.: Huntington Library, 1999), p. 90.

31. "To the People of Sacramento City" (8 August 1850), *Sacramento Illustrated,* pp. 43–46.

32. See "Terrible Riot at Sacramento," *Alta California,* 15 August 1850; "Latest from Sacramento! Cessation of Hostilities," ibid., 16 August 1850); Benjamin Stillman, "Seeking the Golden Fleece," *Overland Monthly,* November 1873, pp. 417–21; Donald Pisani, "Squatter Law in California, 1850–1858," *Western Historical Quarterly* 25 (Autumn 1994): 277–310.

33. For illnesses on the journey to California, see John H. Eagle to Margaret H. Eagle, 10 April 1852, John H. Eagle Correspondence, HUN; for illnesses in the gold country see Samuel Nichols to Sarah Ann Nichols, 7 October 1850, Samuel Nichols Collection, HUN.

34. John Frederick Morse, *History of Sacramento* (Sacramento: Book Collector's Club, 1945), pp. 43–46. For the city's efforts to confront threats to public health, see City Council Minutes, 5, 14, 16, and 20 November and 15 December 1849.

35. J. Roy Jones, *Memories, Men, and Medicine: A History of Medicine in Sacramento, California* (Sacramento: Society for Medical Improvement, 1950), pp. 34–35.

36. According to one municipal waste engineer, the average nineteenth-century urban American annually produced between 300 and 1,200 pounds of ashes, 100 to 180 pounds of organic garbage, and 50 pounds of inorganic rubbish. In 1850, Sacramento's residents thus produced, at a minimum, 1,000 tons of ashes, 350 tons of organic waste, and 175 tons of inorganic waste. See Martin Melosi, "'Out of Sight, Out of Mind': The Environment and Disposal of Municipal Refuse, 1860–1920," *The Historian* 35 (1973): 622.

37. Israel Lord Journal, 20 October 1850, HUN.

38. John D. Unruh, *The Plains Across: The Overland Emigrants and the Trans-Mississippi West, 1840–1860* (Urbana: University of Illinois Press, 1979), p. 403.

39. Charles Rosenberg, *The Cholera Years: The United States in 1832, 1849, and 1866,* 2d ed. (Chicago: University of Chicago Press, 1987), pp. 2–3.

40. Isaac Perkins to Daniel Perkins, 27 October 1850, Isaac Perkins Correspondence.

41. Lord Journal, 23 October 1850.

42. Lord Journal, 23 and 31 October, 6 and 11 November, 22 December 1850; "Sacramento," *Alta California,* 3 November 1850.

43. Eifler, *Gold Rush Capitalists,* pp. 97–100.

44. Thompson and West, *History of Sacramento,* p. 73.

45. *Sacramento Illustrated,* pp. 54–56.

46. City Council Minutes, 23 July 1850.

47. Its significance mirrored that of the city levee in New Orleans, which Ari Kelman has described as a "municipal icon." See Kelman, *A River and Its City,* p. 161. here, as elsewhere, I am indebted to Kelman's work on cities, levees, and ecology.

48. *G. and O. Amy's Marysville Directory* (San Francisco: Monson and Valentine, 1856), pp. 4–7.

49. "Disastrous Visitation! Great Freshet! Breaks in the Levee!" *Alta California,* 8 March 1852; "The Flood! Sacramento Completely Inundated!" ibid., 9 March 1852; "The Overflow," ibid., 10 March 1852; "The Inundation," ibid., 11 March 1852; "State of the Inundation," ibid., 12 March 1852.

50. "Rain," *Sacramento Daily Union,* 13 November 1861; "The American," ibid., 18 November 1861; "Severe on Rats," ibid., 20 November 1861; "Rain in Grass Valley," ibid., 30 November 1861.

51. "Great Rise in the Rivers," *Sacramento Daily Union,* 28 March 1861; "A Great Calamity—Sacramento Deluged," ibid., 10 December 1861.

52. "Mines and Mining," *Marysville Herald,* 27 January 1854; G. H. Mendell, "Report upon a Project to Protect the Navigable Waters of California from the Effects of Hydraulic Mining," H. ex. doc. 98, 47th Cong., 1st Sess. (1882), p. 13; Rossiter Raymond, *Silver and Gold: An Account of Mining and Metallurgical Industry of the United States* (New York: J. B. Ford, 1873), p. 17.

53. W. H. Drum, "Testimony Taken by the Committee on Mining Debris, as Reported to the Assembly," 22d Session, 1877–78. *Appendix to the Journals of the Senate and Assembly of the 22nd Session of the Legislature of the State of California,* vol. 4 (Sacramento: F. P. Thompson, 1878), p. 77.

54. Otto von Geldern, *An Analysis of the Problem of the Proposed Rehabilitation of Hydraulic Mining in California* (Sutter County, 3 January 1928), p. 4.

55. A. T. Arrowsmith, James H. Keyes, J. H. Jewett, and Joseph Johnson, "Testimony Taken by the Committee on Mining Debris," pp. 4–5, 80–82, 100, 105, 141.

56. *James H. Keyes v. Little York Gold Washing and Water Company* (1879), pp. 15–16. N. S. Hanlin, W. H. Drum, "Testimony Taken by the Committee on Mining Debris," pp. 77, 137–38. See also *Address of George Cadwalader, Delivered at Sacramento, February 28 and March 1st, 1882, on the Case of the State of California vs. Gold Run Hydraulic Mining Co.* (Sacramento: H. S. Crocker & Co., 1882), p. 43.

57. Von Geldern, *Hydraulic Mining,* p. 9.

58. "The River," *Sacramento Daily Union,* 21 November 1861; "Improvements," ibid., 26 November 1861; "Board of Supervisors," and "The River," ibid., 29 November 1861; "The Bulkhead," ibid., 30 November 1861; "The River," ibid., 3 December 1861; "The River" and "No Water," ibid., 6 December 1861; "To Be Repaired," ibid. 7 December 1861.

59. "The Flood: Destruction in the Interior," *Sacramento Daily Union,* 11 December 1861; ibid., 13 December 1861.

60. "A Great Calamity—Sacramento Deluged."

61. "A Great Calamity-Sacramento Deluged." "The Flood in Sacramento," *Sacramento Daily Union,* 11 December 1861; "Dead Animals," ibid., 13 December 1861.

62. "The Flooded Portion," *Sacramento Daily Union,* 13 December 1861; "The Rivers," ibid., 1 January 1862; "The Levee Near R Street," ibid., 3 January 1862; "The Condition of the City" and "Levee Repairs," ibid., 4 January 1862; "The Levee Work" and "Railroad Lumber," ibid., 7 January 1862; "Communication with the Interior," ibid., 10 January 1862.

63. "Another Destructive Flood," *Sacramento Daily Union,* 11 January 1862; "Deaths from Drowning" and "The Rise and Fall of the Flood," ibid., 13 January 1862; "Dead Bodies Found," ibid., 14 January 1862; "The Levee at the Tannery," ibid., 21 January 1862; "The Levee at Rabel's Gone," ibid., 23 January 1862; "The Flood," ibid., 24 January 1862.

64. Thompson and West, *History of Sacramento County,* pp. 74–75.

65. William L. Willis, *History of Sacramento County, California* (Los Angeles: Historic Record Company, 1913), p. 116.

7

Fair Play

Outdoor Recreation and Environmental Inequality in Twentieth-Century Seattle

Matthew Klingle

When Caroline Sheldon visited Seattle in 1908, she gushed: "there is perhaps no other city in America which makes such an appeal to the imagination." Despite the city's "apparently chronic condition" of digging, building, and renovating, she found that "the true Seattleite is singularly free from nervousness and worry" because "he appreciates the magnificent scenery and manages to find some time to enjoy it." Countless lakes beckoned swimmers and boaters, and the surrounding "forest primeval" fed lumber mills and the desires of weekend campers alike. Even the "poorest child," she concluded, could "come in contact with nature" here. Seattle's appeal lay in its proximity to the restorative properties of the great outdoors, and the way that people enjoyed this appeal, Sheldon intimated, was as consumers.[1]

Consumer culture has long fascinated historians, and recent studies have followed urban consumers into their workplaces, homes, and shopping malls.[2] In contrast, despite the pathbreaking work of such scholars as William Cronon, environmental historians have seemed uninterested in the urban connections between consumption, social power, and material change. This is a missed opportunity because environmental historians, compared to their peers, pay more attention to the material world that we all devour. Consumption is about status and politics, but it is also about the physical transformations of nature that reorder relationships between producer and consumer across time and space. Yet even what scholars label as productive or consumptive reveals a more complicated history that strikes at the heart of environmentalism. An urban environmental history of consumption might shed light on how conservation (and the environmental movement that followed it) justified certain kinds of consumption in the name of condemning others.[3]

One path toward this more complex history is to connect a salient theme of North American city life—the modern leisure economy—with an ongoing debate within environmental history—the contested landscapes of recreation.[4] Urban historians, especially labor historians, have argued that studying recreation as a form of consumption helps to explain the distinctiveness of the United States working class. In particular, the emergence of mass culture in the early twentieth century, from movie theaters to dance halls, reshaped working-class communities while further segmenting urbanites into discrete groups defined by their consumer preferences. By the postwar period, this new network of consumerism, nurtured by government and business, and endorsed by organized labor, yielded a new landscape of shopping malls and subdivisions for those able to flee decaying industrial cities. Lizabeth Cohen has argued that this "Consumers' Republic" dissolved into a constellation of fragmented and sometimes antagonistic consumer groups by the end of the century.[5]

Environmental historians, in contrast, have largely confined their critiques of consumption and recreation to the struggles between urban sportsmen and the rural residents whose activities they deemed destructive.[6] Indeed, as these scholars have argued, some of the most sacred verities of modern environmentalism, from wilderness to biodiversity, first emerged in the conservation movement as devices to protect certain consumer privileges at the expense of others. Other historians have found that middle-class suburbanites during the 1950s and 1960s helped to launch the environmental movement. Yet the same green-minded citizens rejected alliances with blue-collar neighbors or minorities who suffered the same afflictions of pollution and urban sprawl; in some cases, they even excluded these undesirables from their Arcadian neighborhoods and playgrounds.[7] With the exception of two recent studies on wilderness advocacy and conservation policy, what happened in the intervening years, between the turn of the century and World War II, remains something of a mystery. Paul Sutter analyzes the battle against automobiles encroaching upon wilderness, shedding light on how the anticonsumerist strain of environmental politics got its start, while Kendrick Clements rehabilitates Herbert Hoover as an ardent conservationist who championed outdoor recreation as an antidote to the stresses of modern life.[8]

This essay suggests that there was a complex historical relationship between the new leisure economy and the transformation of urban space in the years before the modern environmental movement, one that encompassed more than debates over wilderness protection and access to public lands. In Seattle, this history began with the rapid physical growth of the city at the turn of the twentieth century. Redirecting rivers, filling estuaries, and building parks completely reworked the landscapes of the city and its environs for the benefit of middle-class outdoor recreation. The production of these new spaces from the late 1890s to the Great Depression generated a new geography of leisure for middle-class Seattleites.[9] Remaking urban space became a process, both material and symbolic, that not only enhanced nature but also enriched society by promoting consumption.

Catching fish and climbing mountains were more than just matters of leisure. They were also matters of politics and power; the new geography of leisure was also a new geography of inequality. As the philosopher Henri Lefebvre argued, "the *right to nature* entered into social practice thanks to *leisure*," and the class that wanted to assert that right most strongly was Seattle's middle class.[10] This influential group reinvented the city's physical environs as a set of segregated spaces dedicated to production and consumption. Productive spaces were set aside for those enterprises essential to progressive urban living, such as manufacturing, retailing, and shipping; consumptive spaces were reserved for those leisure activities that were also essential to progressive urban living, such as fishing, boating, or camping. Production and consumption were thus inscribed into the landscape as complementary, mutually constituting forces, yet in practice the asserted material, social, and cultural distinctions between these activities were fuzzy, the boundaries separating them inherently porous. White-collar professionals, who worked for the city's major businesses as well as Seattle's cultural and political institutions, were the leaders of local conservation groups and the most avid of outdoor enthusiasts. Previous historians have thus neglected a central fact of urban development: recreational users were as active and sometimes as influential in creating spaces for industry and leisure as were the engineers and planners who have dominated urban historiography. The reason was that they shared a common culture of consumption.

And in Seattle, one of the most popular ways to consume was playing outdoors. When middle-class consumers were unable to enforce the spatial distinctions between work and play, conflict erupted. At first, the desire for outdoor recreation in Seattle spanned class divides, but by the Roaring Twenties, it became another front in a larger war over the meaning and uses of urban space. Seattle's outdoor playgrounds became battlegrounds for who had the right to define "work" or "play" in the modern city and its environs. Retreating into the spectacular scenery extolled by Caroline Sheldon did not free Seattleites from worry; it only amplified the anxieties they hoped to flee.

"A Country Full of Charms": Boosting Seattle for Urban Recreation

Selling Seattle to consumers had begun well before Sheldon penned her magazine article. The drive to advertise Seattle's recreational virtues coincided with the full integration of Puget Sound into the national mass market, an integration made possible, in part, by iron and gold. The arrival of the Great Northern Railroad in 1893 and the 1896–1898 Klondike Gold Rush put Seattle on the map. While the Northern Pacific had chosen nearby Tacoma as its terminus in 1887, the Great Northern selected Seattle, creating the city's first transcontinental link. So when George Washington Carmack found gold on the banks of the Klondike River in Canada's Yukon Territory in 1896, Seattle businesses were already well positioned to make a killing. The real profits lay in provisioning the tens of thousands of miners en route to the gold fields. Merchants capitalized upon the miners' need for sturdy shoes, reliable equipment, nonperishable food, accurate guidebooks, and efficient transportation. Many of the city's mercantile giants, such as the famous clothier Nordstrom, got their start by mining the miners thanks to an economic network that stretched from Chicago's stockyards to camps on the Arctic permafrost.[11]

Seattle's political and business leaders realized that gold alone would not sustain their city and set about to turn the landscapes surrounding Seattle into another source of wealth. At the very time that the railroads and the Gold Rush incorporated Seattle into a national, even global mass market, boosters labored to integrate their region's diverse physical environs into the city (map 1). Beginning in the 1890s, civil engineers and city planners rearranged Seattle's topography and hydrology in order to prevent floods, attract industry, eliminate disease, and promote development. They believed building cities completed nature, making it better than before and releasing its regenerative properties to drive social reform. Rather than using nature to rescue the city, these experts saw urbanization as synchronizing culture with environment for the benefit of both.

These transformations unfolded in four interlocking projects that framed how Seattle residents would consume nature through recreation. The first task was to rationalize the boundaries between water and land. At the same time that the Klondike attracted thousands to Seattle, citizens quarreled over how best to drain wetlands, straighten rivers, and fill tidelands. By the beginning of the twentieth century, the path of improvement had been charted. In 1914, city-operated dredges removed the oxbows and meanders of the lower Duwamish River and filled its estuaries, replacing them with wharves and warehouses. To the northwest, the Army Corps of Engineers completed a canal in 1916 connecting freshwater Lake Washington, which hugged Seattle's eastern flank, to Puget Sound, thereby lowering the lake by nearly ten feet. The Cedar River, which drained into the Duwamish at its confluence with the Black River, was redirected to provide Seattle's water supply, with the remainder diverted to flow directly into Lake Washington to provide water for the new canal. In a few years, engineers had changed the plumbing of an entire watershed that once drained forty-one hundred square miles to meet the demand for water, flood control, transportation, and real estate.[12]

The second task was to master the city's rugged topography, the legacy of extensive glacial action in the late Pleistocene. Between 1898 and 1931, city engineers undertook over sixty separate leveling projects, called regrades, that changed the elevation of over twenty major downtown streets and

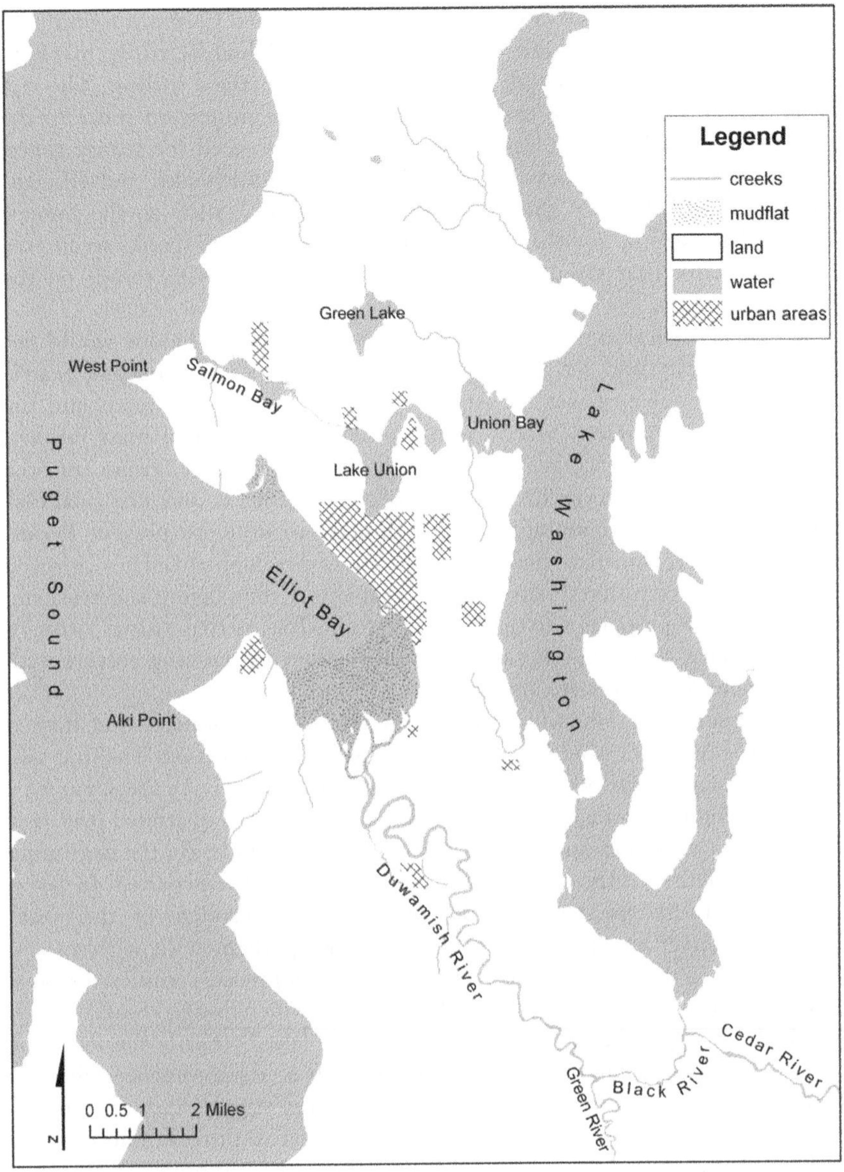

Map 1. Seattle and environs, c. 1890. Map by Amir Sheikh and Matthew Klingle.

removed several large hills. They used pickaxes, steam shovels, and eventually hydraulic cannons to erase the city's mounts, using the earth and rock to fill in tide flats and ravines. Removing hills fed demand for affordable, level land while eradicating habitat for vermin and neighborhoods full of substandard housing.[13]

The third enterprise was to build an urban park system to accentuate the aforementioned improvements. In 1903 the Board of Parks Commissioners hired the Olmsted Brothers, the famed landscape architectural firm, to design and build a network of parks, beaches, and boulevards. While the original plan was scrapped in favor of something more economical, the resulting design was one of the most extensive systems in the urban West. Parks became more than green signifiers of urbanity; they were also public spaces that enhanced property values and promoted civic discourse. By defining Seattle's lack of parks as a problem, the Olmsteds and city officials built distinct spaces for discrete groups such as playgrounds for rambunctious children and arboretums for refined nature lovers.[14] In this fashion, Seattle's business and political elites justified audacious projects because remaking nature harnessed its physical properties to drive social progress (map 2).

The fourth undertaking, claiming a new hinterland for recreation, was more cultural than material at first. Just as railway and business elites touted Seattle's physical advantages to sell its investment prospects, they now extolled the city's environs to justify its lucrative leisure possibilities. Seattle's frontier image could become another engine to generate riches. The Chamber of Commerce crowed in an 1898 pamphlet that Seattle was "a health and pleasure resort of deserved fame" that offered tourists "a country full of charms."[15] The Chamber soon laid claim to Mount Rainier, some seventy miles to the south, as the city's rugged icon, working with the Great Northern and Northern Pacific Railways to help create Mount Rainier National Park in 1899 as a "new pleasuring ground."[16]

Boosters did not stop at the mountain, but also pulled other places, far and near, into the metropolitan orbit of tourism. Selling Seattle reached its apogee at the 1909 Alaska-Yukon-Pacific Exposition, or AYPE, where exhibits and amusements not only celebrated Seattle as the putative gateway to Alaska, Canada, and East Asia, but also proclaimed how city engineers had tirelessly transformed the city to serve as the grand entrance to this land of wealth and beauty.[17] As Welford Beaton, the AYPE's director of publicity, wrote after the exposition: "Nature apparently grew tired before she finished Seattle. She made a wonderful harbor, produced an empire of timber-hung pictures on the horizon, spread three lakes among the hills and then left the town site to itself like a tousled, unmade bed." Only when "Man," Beaton continued, completed "the work which Nature had left undone" could commerce "pour unhampered [into] its natural channels" and begin the real work that nature was intended to do. He gestured to the belief that masculine

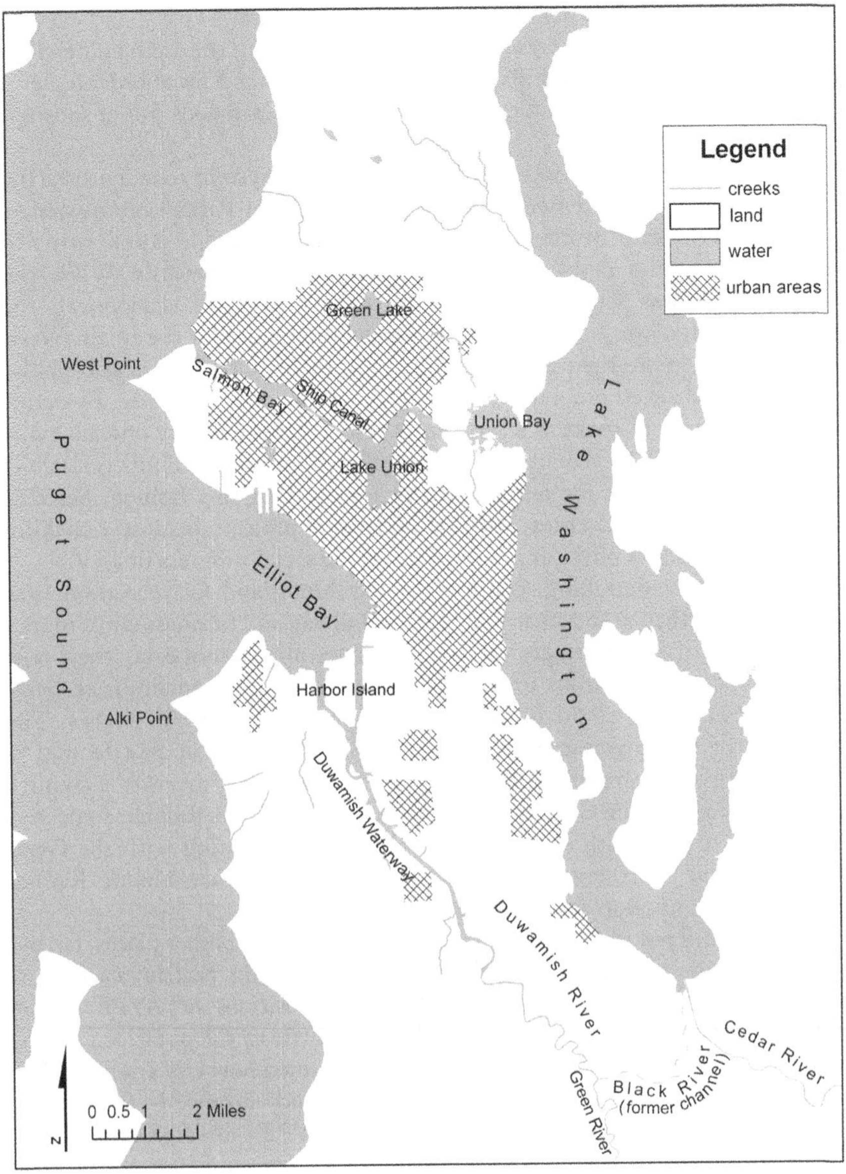

Map 2. Seattle and environs, c. 1920. Map by Amir Sheikh and Matthew Klingle.

engineers gave seminal shape to an incomplete and feminine nature. Not unlike previous world's fairs, from Chicago's 1893 Columbian Exposition to Portland's 1905 Lewis and Clark Exposition, the AYPE exalted this marriage of city to nature.[18]

The 1909 fair also served as a map to this expanded geography of commerce and leisure. Seattle now pulled Alaska, Idaho, Montana, and even Canada's British Columbia and Yukon Territory into its grasp. The Northern Pacific Railway, in its annual travel brochure, *Wonderland,* had ballyhooed the recreational prospects awaiting travelers in the Cascade and Olympic Mountains since the late 1890s, but now local periodicals followed suit, publishing reviews promoting outdoor amusements. One thing that united these "mental territories" was an emphasis upon recreation.[19] Although businesses longed to exploit northern forests and minerals, they also saw the tourists as another resource, since visitors would inevitably pass through town for provisions and transportation just as Klondike miners had done.[20]

Selling this landscape of leisure required new worlds for tourists to experience. Just as city engineers had finished nature for urban growth, tourists and pleasure seekers also enhanced nature even as outdoor recreation rejuvenated them. One Chamber of Commerce pamphlet bragged how human efforts combined with nature to turn all of Seattle into "a magnificent park of unequalled beauty" that made "men stronger, and wiser, and better, which raises them above the weary cares of life and adds largely to the sum total of their happiness."[21] Indeed, happiness and health were the very beings that inhabited this refined landscape. Zoë Kincaid wrote in the *Seattle Mail and Herald* in 1905 how Seattleites lived as perpetual vacationers, building "inns in the mountains and on the bays and inlets of the Sound." Even those "people of moderate means" could "enjoy the woods or water" and watch their children grow "straight as pines, learned in water craft and wood lore." "Brought up in the shadows of the mountains," Seattle's youth were "taught to be true Westerners, men and women of right-living and thinking."[22]

By marketing its hinterland as a recreational paradise, Seattle emulated New York City and Boston in their appropriation of the Adirondacks, Berkshires, and rural northern New England.[23] The difference was that Seattle boosters could seamlessly integrate city and countryside in their campaigns as part of a "Charmed Land" or an "Evergreen Playground" thanks to new media and transportation technologies. Railway agents made this message part of their "See America First" campaign, with one circular proclaiming: "Here you will play harder, with more zest and enjoyment" because "you can't help to do it. . . . *Everyone* does out here!"[24] Promoters stressed that the Northwest appealed to would-be rusticators and sophisticated urban vacationers alike. "Lest you form a mental picture of this great vacation play land as a vast and lovely wilderness," Great Northern Railroad promoters cautioned, "there are the cities." Seattle in particular was modern, up-to-date, and clean. And, most important, it was consumer-friendly, full of stores, theaters, and other amusements. "One can so delightfully 'gad about,'" the authors continued, because "there is a decided satisfaction in knowing that one has such a wealth of riches from which to choose as one may please." In the pages of booster pamphlets, Seattle seemed more like a giant department store or mail order catalogue than an actual city.[25]

Boosting Seattle's recreational opportunities was about inventing and selling new experiences for urbanites to consume. It was a method to convince visitors and longtime residents that city and nature yielded endless diversions as well as economic security and social stability. Playing in the outdoors was more than an idle pursuit. It was also central to how reformers envisioned the role of nature in promoting a civic commonwealth of leisure and consumption.

"Our Childhood Geographies Come True": Reform and Reaction in the Playtime City

As the editors of *Welfare: The Journal of Municipal and Social Progress,* a Seattle monthly, wrote in 1913, "play is as important as work." Without the "play instinct," the editors warned, "one of the forces that have led men into the wilderness and hence to the discovery and conquest of new lands" would disappear. Play was the only way to achieve "the blending together of the whole man." The editors of *Welfare* had encapsulated an important premise of twentieth-century American life—the therapeutic society—and how it intersected with the environmental history of the city. Urban reformers from London to San Francisco had long worried that modern cities were literally killing people. At first, their attention focused on the material manifestations of urbanization—poor sanitation, disease, and pollution—but their attention soon turned toward reforming civic character as well. The genesis of consumption as cultural complaint grew from the feeling among bourgeois urbanites that Americans, especially men, had become "over-civilized" and needed to live, as Theodore Roosevelt had done, a more strenuous life. Living in a machine-made world, white-collar manager and blue-collar worker alike had become obsessed with finding "the real thing" through recreation.[26]

The quest to rediscover nature through play began as Seattleites of all classes threw themselves into vigorous outdoor pursuits. As Almira Bailey announced in the Chamber of Commerce booklet *Seattle and the Charmed Land,* the "Puget Sound Region of the Pacific Northwest is our childhood geographies come true." Bicycling, hunting, fishing, and camping all became wildly popular, with daily newspapers listing routes, advertising equipment, and pushing for improved access.[27] The physical distance between city and country was shrinking in turn-of-the-century America as interurban railways, then automobile roads, made the countryside more accessible. Organizations such as the Washington State Good Roads Association, founded in 1899, aggressively lobbied county and state officials for more and better thoroughfares. In turn, social scientists, such as Norman Hayner, noted how automobile camping paid dividends for local businesses.[28] At the same time, what historian Peter Schmitt called "literary commuters" also telescoped the distance between metropolis and hinterland.[29] One prolific literary commuter in Seattle was W. S. Phillips, a local sportswriter who went by the romantic pseudonym "El Comancho" and publicized Seattle's "new Garden of Eden." "By all means," he crowed, "if you live in the old, staid, provincial East, pack your suit bags some day . . . and find out what living really means." Phillips saw profit in outdoor recreation, and like other boosters, he realized that attracting tourists meant attracting future residents who shared a passion for the outdoors—and would be willing to pay to play.[30]

Boosters like Phillips realized that outdoor recreation had an important role in promoting reform and progress. Outdoor clubs such as the Mountaineers simultaneously endorsed wilderness sports while advancing particular social aims (figure 1). Based upon similar societies in other west coast cities—the Mazamas of Portland and the Sierra Club of San Francisco—the Mountaineers, formed in 1906, tapped members of Seattle's interlocking commercial and reformist circles. Founders included photographer and Chamber of Commerce leader Asahel Curtis (brother of the famed photographer and chronicler of the American Indian Edward S. Curtis), electrical magnate W. Montelius Price, and University of Washington history professor Edmond S. Meany. By 1907, the club had 233 members enthusiastic "to explore the mountains, forests and water courses of the Pacific Northwest." Meany, who served as president for twenty-seven years, claimed to speak for the Mountaineers when promoting Seattle, and vice versa. Curtis did the same. In many respects, the early Mountaineers behaved like the urban boosters they were.[31]

Even when they were in the back country, the Mountaineers could not escape their predilection for reform. The club was, at first, primarily a social venture for participants who took mountain hikes, dressed in Sunday finery, and spent the night at a rustic cabin near Snoqualmie Pass for banquets, dancing, avant garde plays, and poetry readings. The centerpiece of the Mountaineers' social agenda was the annual summer outing, which drew as many as one hundred participants charged to bring packs filled with required equipment and follow a long list of rules. Enforcing military-like discipline was necessary, in part, to save lives. As Curtis wrote in his report of the first outing in 1907, strict adherence to club rules prevented tragedy when inclement weather drove back an attempt to climb ice-clad Mount Olympus. While the Mountaineers rhapsodized about the freedom of the hills, they also brought industrial efficiency with them for very practical, consumer-minded reasons.[32] When they were not traipsing up mountainsides, the Mountaineers

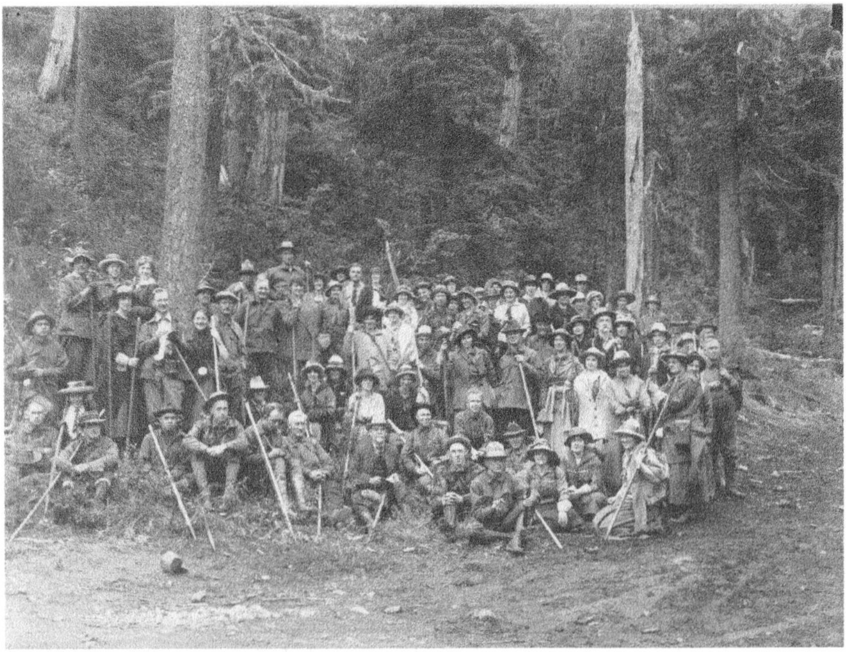

Figure 1. Mountaineers group photo in the Cascades, c. 1920. Museum of History and Industry, Seattle, MOHAI 93.16.20.2.

worked to catalogue all of Washington's back-country trails while building new ones so "that those who follow may find and enjoy the same beauties." Rules and work parties were part of a larger mission to inculcate common standards for playing in nature.[33]

Just as reform imperatives guided the Mountaineers, they also affected other organizations that used outdoor recreation to promote social change. In response to the Mountaineers' exclusiveness and strict adherence to rules, disaffected wilderness aficionados formed the Co-Operative Campers in 1916 to "make our mountains accessible through co-operative camps and to encourage a love of simple living in the open air."[34] The Co-op Campers also organized summer expeditions and local walks, promoted conservation ethics, and taught good camping skills. Unlike the Mountaineers, they did not require members to purchase their gear or indulge in expensive get-togethers. Instead, members pooled their money to acquire tents, sleeping bags, packs, and food collectively (figure 2). Membership fees stayed at one dollar, and anyone could join if they could prove their mettle as capable camper.[35] Most members were trade unionists and full-time industrial workers, with a smattering of bohemians and radicals. This was leisure with an ideological edge.

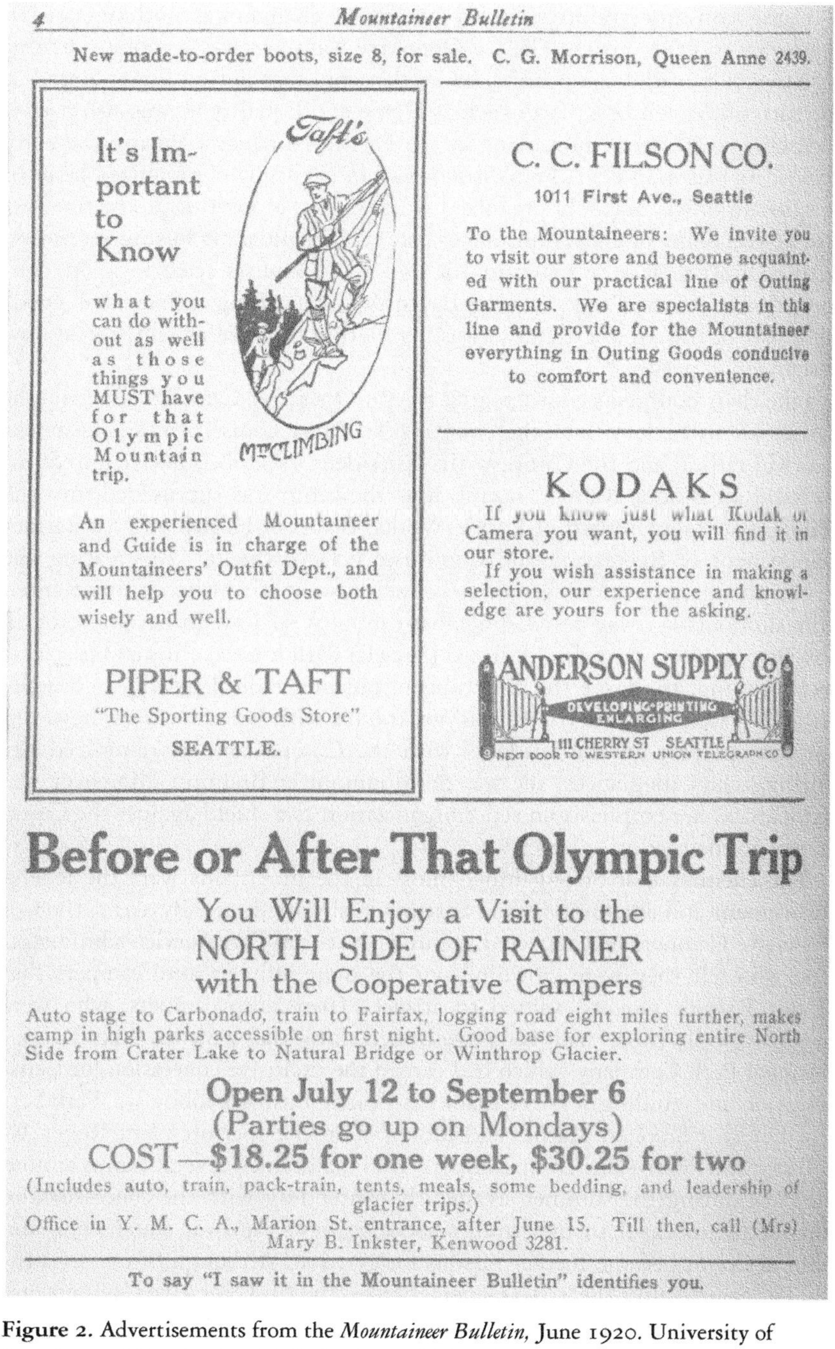

4 *Mountaineer Bulletin*

New made-to-order boots, size 8, for sale. C. G. Morrison, Queen Anne 2439.

It's Important to Know

what you can do without as well as those things you MUST have for that Olympic Mountain trip.

An experienced Mountaineer and Guide is in charge of the Mountaineers' Outfit Dept., and will help you to choose both wisely and well.

PIPER & TAFT

"The Sporting Goods Store"

SEATTLE.

C. C. FILSON CO.

1011 First Ave., Seattle

To the Mountaineers: We invite you to visit our store and become acquainted with our practical line of Outing Garments. We are specialists in this line and provide for the Mountaineer everything in Outing Goods conducive to comfort and convenience.

KODAKS

If you know just what Kodak or Camera you want, you will find it in our store.

If you wish assistance in making a selection, our experience and knowledge are yours for the asking.

ANDERSON SUPPLY Co

DEVELOPING-PRINTING ENLARGING

111 CHERRY ST SEATTLE

NEXT DOOR TO WESTERN UNION TELEGRAPH CO

Before or After That Olympic Trip

You Will Enjoy a Visit to the

NORTH SIDE OF RAINIER

with the Cooperative Campers

Auto stage to Carbonado, train to Fairfax, logging road eight miles further, makes camp in high parks accessible on first night. Good base for exploring entire North Side from Crater Lake to Natural Bridge or Winthrop Glacier.

Open July 12 to September 6

(Parties go up on Mondays)

COST—$18.25 for one week, $30.25 for two

(Includes auto, train, pack-train, tents, meals, some bedding, and leadership of glacier trips.)

Office in Y. M. C. A., Marion St. entrance, after June 15. Till then, call (Mrs) Mary B. Inkster, Kenwood 3281.

To say "I saw it in the Mountaineer Bulletin" identifies you.

Figure 2. Advertisements from the *Mountaineer Bulletin,* June 1920. University of Washington Libraries, Special Collections, UW23989z.

Using consumer politics to advance social change was nothing new in Seattle or in other cities. The Co-Operative Campers was a mobile, urban-based version of the communitarian settlements that dotted Puget Sound at the turn of the century, places such as Home and Equality. It was also part of a vibrant cooperative movement in the Pacific Northwest during the early 1900s. As historian Dana Frank discovered in her study of organized labor in Seattle, unionists not only organized workers at the point of production but also at the point of consumption to foster class solidarity. Fusing recreation with radicalism was an extension of the how unionists tried to make consumption a political act. Staging boycotts and pushing union label goods were part of this strategy, and so was instructing blue-collar campers on how best to enjoy nature.[36]

Like their bourgeois counterparts, the Co-Operative Campers also brought the urban with them into the countryside. Anna Louise Strong, the noted political radical and the Campers' first president, described one trip to Summerland on Mount Rainier, noting how the camp was subdivided into the "Fire Department, Board of Public Works, Board of Health and Sanitation, Department of Recreation and Commissary Department." Re-creating the city in an alpine meadow seemed to be inconsistent with what Strong wanted from outdoors—a way to rebel against capitalist society. In her autobiography, Strong wrote that she "drugged [herself] with forests, cliffs and glaciers" every summer to escape the afflictions of pushing radical politics in Seattle. Strong's affinity for orderliness was not at odds with her radicalism, however. For one, playing in the outdoors with the Co-op Campers reinforced her working-class allegiances; she was no Mountaineer Brahmin. Moreover, she rationalized her emphasis on strict organization as a shield against the Co-op Campers' enemies.[37]

The enemies that Strong feared most in the mountains were the federal government and anti-unionists in Seattle's business cliques. By 1917, the Co-Operative Campers had attracted the ire of National Park Service administrators, who felt they were crowding out the more affluent auto campers that Mount Rainier rangers wanted to attract. These auto campers, who were largely middle-class, had been welcomed into the park by the Rainier National Park Company, which had earned the exclusive concession for transportation and guiding services thanks to Seattle business lobbyists. Park Service Director Stephen Mather and Mount Rainier Superintendent Roger W. Toll saw the lower-class Co-op campers, who maintained several camps around the park during the summer, as unfairly contending with the concessionaire and sought to expel them. Strong's socialist views, antiwar statements, and labor activism became further reasons for eviction. Although Strong eventually left Seattle after the 1919 General Strike, the Co-Operative Campers and the Park Service continued to clash until 1922, when the Campers disbanded and disappeared. Despite their rivalry, however, the Co-Operative Campers and the Mountaineers, which seemed like natural antagonists, cooperated to open Mount Rainier for public camping. Employing protests, hearings, and letter-writing campaigns, both organizations forced the Park Service to build free campgrounds and ended the monopoly of the Rainier National Park Company by the end of the 1920s. Meany and Strong, enemies on almost every other issue, agreed that camping on public lands was a consumer right worth protecting.[38]

The decline of the cooperative camping movement in the Pacific Northwest did not spell an end to alternative visions of urban-based outdoor recreation, but it did channel them into tracks where profits and affordability trumped class allegiances. Seattle's now-famous Recreational Equipment Cooperative, Incorporated, or REI, was the best example of the new trend. Lloyd Anderson, REI's founder, was a member of the Mountaineers but rebelled at having to attend chic parties. In 1937, Anderson staged a coup d'état just two years after Meany died, ousted the old guard, and helped to install leaders focused more on strenuous sports, such as rock climbing. Anderson did more than remake the Mountaineers; he also transformed how its members bought their requisite equipment. Influenced by his participation in several Seattle co-ops, Anderson and his climbing partners organized REI in 1939. By pooling members' annual membership fees and ordering materials collectively from Europe, Anderson was able to purchase high-quality equipment at affordable prices. He soon won loyal customers nationwide. Yet REI was a faint shadow of the Co-op Campers; it espoused the ideals of collective action, but only to deploy them in the pursuit of individual consumption.[39]

Outdoor recreation had now become both a way of life and a business for many Seattle residents as the rising power of mass consumption began to reshape urban life across the United States. Sociologists Robert and Helen Merrill Lynd noticed this phenomenon in their classic 1929 study, *Middletown,* as they observed the effects of the automobile, motion pictures, radio, and mass advertising upon urban recreation. The demand for quality goods to help people play, the Lynds concluded, drove manufacturers to make better products.[40]

Seattle became a seedbed for sporting goods innovation, and entrepreneurs such as Eddie Bauer took advantage of consumer desires for equipment now seen as essential for enjoyable outings. But unlike Lloyd Anderson and Anna Louise Strong, Bauer had no pretensions of protest; he was a capitalist first. Born on Orcas Island in northern Puget Sound, Bauer had worked in several Seattle sporting goods stores before opening his own shop in 1920. He consciously catered to the city's middle- and upper-class outdoorsmen, selling hand-tied steelhead flies and his patented line of down sleeping bags and jackets. Bauer also relentlessly advertised the region's fishing and hunting opportunities, working with friends and fishing buddies at the *Seattle Times* and the Chamber of Commerce. After weekend trips, he would proudly display his trophies—strings of glistening trout and salmon, heads of deer and elk—in front of his downtown store (figure 3). And through his mail-order catalogues and retail outlet, filled with images of hunters and fishermen pursuing their quarry through tall trees and snowy peaks, Bauer sold the Northwest's outdoors lifestyle to consumers across the country.[41]

The business of teaching and selling outdoor sports was also the business of municipal agencies thanks to the "back to nature" movement sweeping across urban America. Reformers worried that city children had "lost all manner of vestigial activities, hunting and fishing, climbing and swimming and exploring" crucial to proper juvenile development. In response, educators began teaching children about nature as a way to rescue them from becoming overcivilized.[42] Seattle government agencies followed these trends by using Seattle's great outdoors as a classroom. Public schools launched a gardening program in 1913 to promote the Americanization of Japanese and Italian immigrant children while providing a new "vocational [and] recreational outlook . . . and social service to the community."[43] At the same time, Seattle's Parks Department opened public beaches at Green Lake, Alki Point, and Lake Washington. By the late 1920s, the Department expanded its role to offer swimming and sailing instruction, rowing competitions, day camping for children, snow skiing at Snoqualmie Pass, and still more municipal playgrounds and beaches. An automobile camp at Woodland Park, opened in 1922, attracted nearly twelve thousand visitors annually within two years of its opening. The Parks Department now considered outdoor recreation its top priority.[44]

This shift toward state-sponsored recreation was part of a nationwide trend in the 1920s that connected leisure and consumption to Americanism. Secretary of Commerce Herbert Hoover summarized this synthesis in a 1924 letter to the National Parks Association, accepting the presidency of the organization. "Recreation grounds and natural museums are as necessary to advancing our civilization," he maintained, "as are wheat fields and factories." As an engineer, Hoover believed that technocratic elites could build cultural contentment and social unity for Americans just as they had manufactured material abundance.[45] Hoover's comments resonated in Seattle, a city accustomed to seeing outdoor work and outdoor play as two sides of the same coin. "Seattle makes no mistake in promoting and encouraging all kinds of clean and healthful sports," the Board of Park Commissioners stated in 1922, "and for every dollar invested in the common stock of recreation we get dividends of health, strength, alertness, good behavior, obedience, clean habits, or in a word, good citizenship."[46] City park officials worked with local clubs, such as the Mountaineers, and retailers, such as Eddie Bauer and REI, to maintain facilities, provide instruction, and reinforce voluntarism as the best way to get outside and become more American.[47]

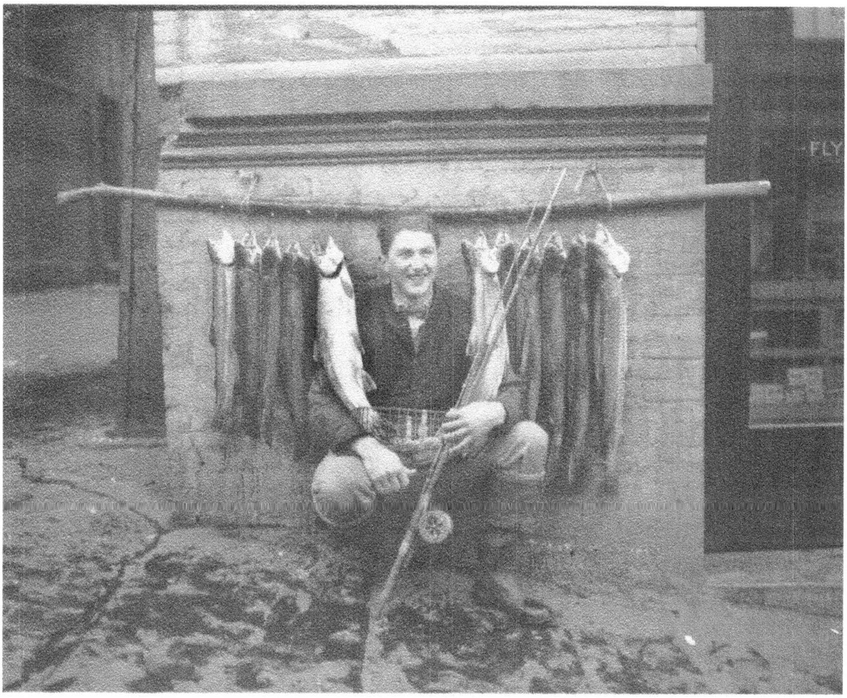

Figure 3. Eddie Bauer in front of his downtown Seattle store with steelhead trout, 1926. Museum of History and Industry, Seattle, MOHAI 83.10.3,109.1.

As Seattleites came to see recreation as an integral part of their daily lives, they required ever more spaces in which to play. In 1927 the Seattle Parks Department started pushing for a new Metropolitan Park District to encompass most of King County. Edmond Meany was enlisted in this effort and two years later, he gave an address titled "The Coming City of Puget Sound." Automobiles and railways, Meany argued, had led to "the contraction of space," so that "the whole Puget Sound region" was a "single contact area from the standpoint of work and play." Only by acquiring more "open spaces" could Seattle meet future recreation demands.[48]

By the 1920s, the dream of greater Seattle advanced at the Alaska-Yukon-Pacific Exposition had come of age. Seattle's recreational hinterland had increased as its citizens' appetite for leisure had grown. School gardens and parks were physical and cultural manifestations of the rural within the urban, while scenic highways and hiking trips took the city and its habits into the countryside. What Meany failed to emphasize was how this integrated landscape of city and countryside was the work of largely middle-class, white professionals who framed outdoor recreation in terms of individual consumption and challenged those who espoused an alternative vision, particularly those who were poorer and less powerful than Meany and his Mountaineers. To even see this landscape depended very much on seeing it through the eyes of the well-off.

"Putting the Small Men Out of Business": Outdoor Recreation and Social Conflict

Although boosters extolled the integration of industry with leisure, the fall-out from merging the two spread across Seattle like ashes from a camper's fire. The benefits settled on those who sailed on Lake Washington, hiked on Mount Rainier, picnicked amidst the pines of Volunteer Park, or fished in Elliott Bay. They believed they were living in a garden city designed for their pleasure. Seattle reflected the unity of work and relaxation in their lives. But if you turned to look at those who lived on boats instead of sailing on them, who used parks for collecting food instead of dining in them, or who caught fish for subsistence or profit instead of for fun, the marvelous landscape of boosters' gazetteers and broadsides went up in smoke. By the 1920s, the quest for playing in the outdoors had become an instrument to expel the working poor from Arcadian playgrounds for the affluent.

The first rifts opened along the city's waterfront and around its remade watershed. Some observers had foreseen how changing Seattle's rivers and lakes would do more than modify the physical landscape; it would transform residents' behaviors as well. Major Hiram Chittenden, the Army Corps of Engineers officer who built the Lake Washington Ship Canal, expressed these sentiments best in 1910. Responding to critics who feared that the canal would ruin Lake Washington, Chittenden replied that the lake would remain "the chief scenic attraction of the city." He concluded that the canal was "a case where utilitarian ends can be accomplished without any sacrifice of sentimental interests."[49] Chittenden spoke from his experience as the primary road surveyor for Yellowstone National Park, and his remarks proved prophetic. Just as automobiles opened national parks to city-weary Americans, affordable motorized launches opened marine and fresh waters to weekend explorers. Prior to the canal's opening in 1916, a reporter for *Pacific Motor Boat,* a monthly magazine, remarked that Seattle would soon have "both a land and water system of highways" that would make the city both useful and beautiful.[50] Afterwards, weekend mariners became the canal's most avid users.

As Chittenden had predicted, the Ship Canal had opened up a scenic waterscape that some also considered their home. Class differences marked the divergent types of houseboats that clustered along the city's remade lakes and rivers. Ramshackle tubs on Lake Union and the Duwamish Waterway housed Seattle's itinerant laborers who wanted cheap, temporary dwellings close to jobs in the shipyards and marine shops.[51] By contrast, the houseboaters along Lake Washington were not poor "water gypsies" but the "'Poseidons' and the 'Uranians' of the 'Queen City'" (figure 4). Some were temporary summer homes; others housed "Bohemians" year-round, attracting the admiration of those frightened by the city's tenements. One reporter quipped: "if the city's soulless populations prefer stuffy apartments to the airy houseboats," the boaters in Lake Washington had "a taste of liberty and a breath of the free, open, outdoor life."[52]

Those living in houseboats along the Duwamish Waterway soon became embroiled in a conflict sparked by those who wanted to defend the "free, open, outdoor life" from low-class interlopers. Houseboats along the Duwamish housed many of Seattle's commercial fishermen, who migrated between work in Alaska, Puget Sound, and the Columbia River. Most were immigrants from southern and eastern Europe or East Asia; others were Native Americans, living and working off-reservation. When they fished close to home, in the Duwamish and Elliott Bay, they angered wealthier sport anglers who feared their outdoor fun was at risk.

Establishing the original contours of the Duwamish fisheries is difficult, but evidence points to once thriving runs that compared favorably to other major fisheries in Washington. An 1896 survey by the U.S. Fish Commission noted significant populations of coho (silver), chum, and Chinook salmon; they also noted the presence of nonmigratory sockeye salmon (kokanee or redfish) in Lake Washington. Until the 1880s, Seattle stood at the nexus of a productive commercial fishery, but by the end of the century, most fishermen had migrated north to the larger runs on the Fraser River in British Columbia or coastal Alaska. Nonetheless, many still plied the Duwamish and Elliott Bay for the burgeoning local fresh fish market in Seattle.[53]

By the first decades of the twentieth century, the Duwamish runs were in trouble. Salmon fisheries in urban Puget Sound were now on technological life support because state fisheries managers had to provide ever more fish to ever more consumers. State officials turned to hatcheries as natural spawning habitats disappeared. The upper Cedar River had been dammed in 1900 to provide water for Seattle, and dredging to build the Duwamish Waterway removed not only snags and brush but also the gravelly beds and eel grass that were essential spawning habitat. Diverting Lake Washington to spill through the Ship Canal forced salmon that spawned in the lower Cedar and Sammamish Rivers to adopt an entirely new and confusing migration route. Sea gulls preyed upon stunned juveniles that spilled over the locks on their seaward migration; sea lions feasted on returning adults stuck below the locks. And everywhere, pollution fouled waterways, killing adults and offspring alike. Urban anglers began to object and the Washington Department of Fish and Game, bowing to political pressure, built

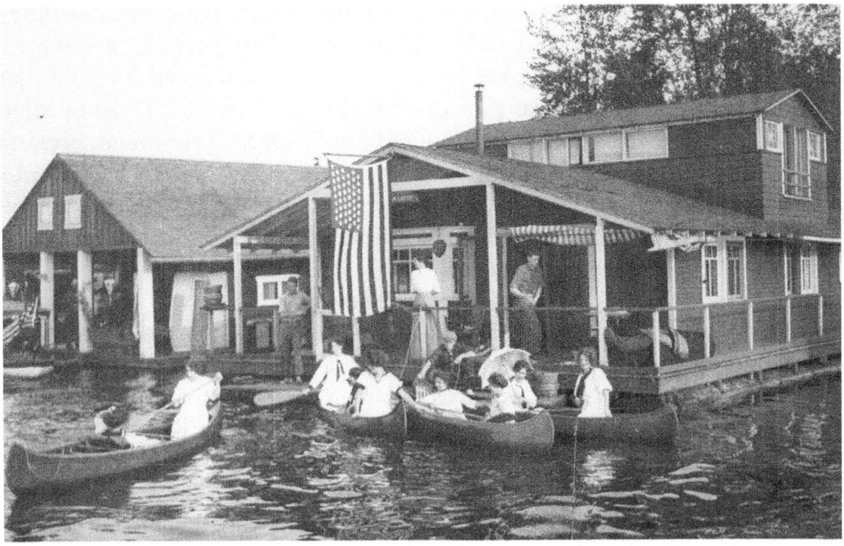

Figure 4. Weekend pleasure houseboats on Lake Washington, 1912. University of Washington Libraries, Special Collections, Lee 20035.

hatcheries along the Duwamish and Green Rivers, as well as along the remaining tributaries to Lake Washington, to mitigate the dismemberment of the original watershed.[54]

Hatcheries were only a partial solution and their mixed effectiveness prompted sportsmen to find the real culprits. The most visible scapegoats were remaining commercial fishers along the Duwamish Waterway. In contrast to their foes, most sport fishers were middle-class, native-born, and politically connected. With the outbreak of World War I, their desires for an unobstructed recreational fishery converged with shippers' wishes for increased maritime traffic. Tugboat operators, shipbuilders, and lumber mills complained in nativist terms how nets and fish traps became entangled in propellers and damaged barges. As W. T. Isted of the Northwestern Tow Boat Owners' Association claimed, most offenders were "ignorant of the English language, or at least they profess to be as they do not pay any attention to the navigation laws of our country."[55] Spatial politics made strange bedfellows. Both groups saw the Duwamish Waterway and Elliott Bay as exclusive, but their rhetoric fell back on the familiar mantra of public access. To preserve waterways as public required recasting them as under attack by special interests. As a result, the lines between work and leisure, production and consumption became hopelessly entangled.[56]

Unable and unwilling to unseat industry or restrict sports anglers, officials decided to oust the commercial fishermen instead. State Fish Commissioner

L. H. Darwin, who was also waging war against commercial and subsistence Indian fishing throughout the state, blamed aliens, mostly "Austrians, principally from the province of Dalmatia, and other southeastern European peoples," for unsustainable fishing. Purse seines and gill nets, popular technology among immigrant fishers on Puget Sound because of their high degree of effectiveness and low cost, were singled out for their pernicious effects. With the most productive hatchery on Puget Sound located just twelve miles upstream from Elliott Bay at Soos Creek, a tributary of the Green and Duwamish Rivers, the health of the region's fisheries was at risk. "The greatest mistake of all," Darwin concluded in his 1917–19 biennial report, "is permitting aliens not only to completely monopolize our fishery, but to permit them to destroy it while monopolizing it." His rhetoric played well against the backdrop of wartime patriotism. Expelling immigrants, who had no legal claim to the fisheries, was easier than expelling industrial interests, who could fall back upon property claims and legal standing.[57]

State officials responded to the rising crescendo of protests by ousting commercial fishers. Nearly six hundred Seattle residents sent petitions to Governor Louis F. Hart in January 1920, claiming that commercial net fishing on the Duwamish deprived "thousands of citizens of both healthful recreation and food" while threatening "the natural propagation of salmon" assisted by the "State hatchery located thereon."[58] After seasonal closures beginning in 1918, the State Fish Commission eventually closed the Duwamish River and Elliott Bay to commercial fishing altogether in February 1920 as well as Shilshole Bay, at the mouth of the Ship Canal. One grateful sportsman thanked the governor and Commission for taking "an interest in our welfare."[59]

Commercial fishers did not surrender without a fight; they attacked their new nemesis, urban sport anglers, and their litany of lament was a contradictory critique of urban overconsumption. On the one hand, farmers and city dwellers took too much water from the Green and Duwamish rivers, leaving too little for the fish at the state salmon hatchery downstream. With insufficient water, spawning salmon could not overcome bars, snags, and other obstacles downstream from the hatchery collection racks. On the other hand, immigrant fishers also defended their work as patriotic, falling back on the rhetoric of producer ideology as their claim to American identity. "Any honest man who wants to work in any lawful pursuit to produce the things that are needed by the people," one group of petitioners argued, should "have an opportunity to do so." Some, like R. Q. Hall, deflected blame to other users. Closing the Duwamish, he shouted at a June 1921 State Fisheries Board hearing, was only "putting the small men out of business" without doing anything to punish the ultimate culprits. Board Chairman E. A. Sims brushed off Hall's protest, yelling back that the Duwamish would never be "opened again in his lifetime."[60]

With legal access now closed to commercial net fishers, poaching emerged as an alternative claim to the Duwamish and Elliott Bay fisheries. Fish thievery was a form of what Karl Jacoby has called "environmental banditry," and arrest records of the State Fish Commissioner outlined the path to conflict. According to the 1925–27 biennial Department of Fisheries report, wardens arrested fourteen separate individuals for net fishing in the Duwamish River. Totals were similar for the rest of the decade as well. Most of those charged with illegal fishing had Italian, Greek, Slavic, or Japanese surnames; some were likely Indians, too.[61]

With local commercial fishing practically eliminated, consumer rhetoric supplanted producer rhetoric in depictions of Seattle's fishing delights. Eddie Bauer extolled in 1928 how "Seattle fishermen are fortunate to have at their very door the finest salt water fishing in the country." "Calvin Coolidge would laugh out loud," the *Seattle Times* stated in 1929, "if he ever caught a Chinook like they haul in by the boatload in Seattle waters." H. L. Dilaway, another local sport fisher, asked rhetorically in 1932 if there was another place where someone could "catch salmon off the docks, or under the shadow of a skyscraper?"[62]

Fisheries scientists and managers helped to perpetuate this image by using artificial propagation to supplement natural runs even as urban demand for outdoor recreation and utilities further imperiled salmon survival. City officials allowed sport anglers to build a small hatchery at Seward Park in 1934, while the State Department of Fisheries built another salmon hatchery in 1936 on Issaquah Creek, a tributary of Lake Sammamish and Lake Washington. State fisheries managers also planted sockeye salmon in Lake Washington, first in 1919, then periodically beginning in 1937, hoping to start a brand new fishery there.[63] One motivation behind expanding hatcheries was that Seattle leaders were unwilling to breach dams on the Cedar River, the city's water source, or the Skagit River, its major electrical generator, in order to save salmon. Such actions only burnished the myth of the commons pervasive to urban sport anglers' faith in unrestricted recreational fishing. What was once public had become private; what was once a fishery for production was now a fishery for recreation where salmon were akin to consumer goods manufactured for individual consumption.[64]

Just as wild salmon had become an industrial product for middle-class sport anglers, Seattle's famed Olmsted-designed parks were becoming another consumer good segmented by race and class. During the 1920s, Audubon Society members inveighed against songbird hunting in city parks, calling for restrictions against aliens, primarily Italian men who used "snares and traps" and Japanese boys who used "air guns [and] sling shots on birds with some effect." These foreign-born hunters, who were "generally ignorant of the game laws and restrictions," were guilty of "indiscriminate shooting" to supply their larders and the illicit feather trade.[65] Opposition to illegal hunting was spatial as well as ideological. Audubon activists emphasized how the worst offenses took place around the shores of Lake Washington, where the lowered water table had produced new wetlands habitat, or in city parks, which housed the remnants of the forests that once covered Seattle. Audubon members were oddly sympathetic to native white residents who trapped nonnative quail, arguing that it was not only "to be expected" but served to eliminate an invasive species.[66]

In an inversion of the Olmstedian ideal, parks had become places where social differences hardened, not softened, through contact among citizens. Along Lake Washington Boulevard, which ran through the wealthy neighborhoods of Mount Baker Park and Madrona, uncouth drivers drove locals to distraction. Ella B. Rowntree grumbled that picnickers were destroying the "pure beauty" of the "natural woodland, flowers, and ferns" along the parkway. "We, who own property surrounding this Park," she continued, "must build and maintain homes of a certain standard in order that this district shall be a desirable and attractive place in which to live." Other high-class districts of Seattle suffered as well. Sigrid M. Frisch railed against low-class visitors dumping "mattresses, bedding, clothing; parts of autos, furnaces, heating leads and packing materials . . . by the auto-loadful" in the ravines below picturesque Queen Anne Boulevard.[67] Seattleites had discovered that the roads they took to the outdoors ran two ways, and by the 1920s, the auto camp in Woodland Park had become an eyesore where campers pitched tents festooned "with lines of washed clothing hung out to dry"(figure 5). Park Board President A. S. Kerry closed the camp in 1929, citing waning attendance and angry neighbors. He justified his decision by arguing "that no more disgusting spectacle was ever exhibited in any city in America than what was brought about by the allotment of space in one of our most beautiful parks to non-resident campers whose primitive, unsanitary living conditions were much worse than they are in the slums of our largest cities."[68]

In a parallel to growing opposition to building roads in national parks, cars were now seen by Seattle park officials as infernal vehicles that violated nature. Kerry's concerns drove efforts to create a Metropolitan Park District to encompass most of King County. "We must not have the unsightly back yard features," he said in a 1928 letter to city voters, "such as camping places, swamps, tin cans and wash tubs placed in parks in the city or in parks close enough to the city so as to destroy the very thing that we are trying to accomplish." Changes intended to beautify city landscapes had failed, tempting the lawless and indigent to colonize them, as they had in Woodland Park or along the Duwamish River. The solution was to build beyond the city. Voters feared additional taxes, however, and rejected the proposal in a special 1929 election. Afterwards, Kerry left the Parks Department in disgust, fearing that Seattle's parks were sliding into permanent decline.[69]

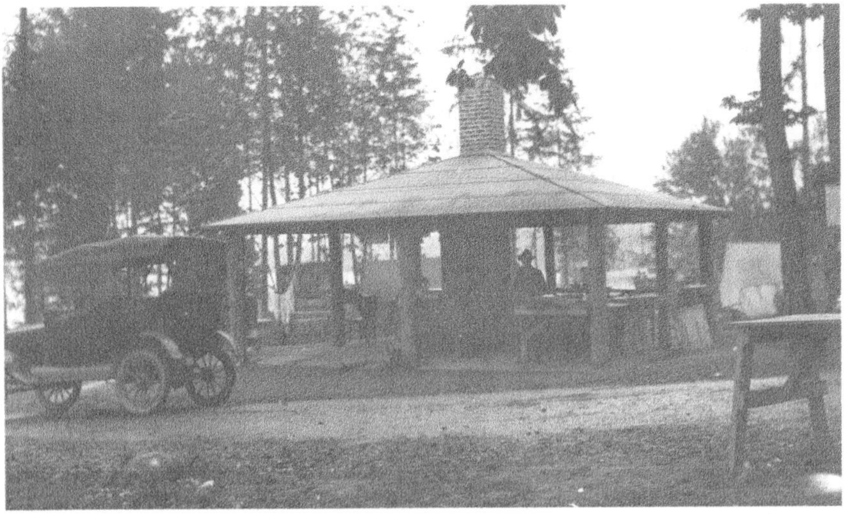

Figure 5. Auto camp at Woodland Park, c. 1925. Seattle Municipal Archives, Photograph Collection, Item 30812.

By the 1930s, it seemed as if Seattle had abandoned the Olmstedian ideal of merging city and nature into a pastoral middle ground. Everywhere the urban garden seemed to be in retreat and the moneyed classes blamed city officials and Seattle's poor for the mess. The city had long used unemployed laborers to build and maintain its parks. During the Great Depression, the Parks Department, with the help of the federal Works Progress Administration, expanded its program. Parks officials often let the poor keep the cut wood from tree and brush removal and stay afterwards for picnics or camping (figure 6). As the Park Board stated in its 1934 report, "Seattle's parks have truly been a godsend to the 'Unemployed' during these past extremely trying years, and have provided practically the only recreation possible to hundreds of people."[70] Parks officials congratulated themselves for providing welfare, but nearby residents saw destruction instead of charity. Passions ran especially high in Seward Park, located at the end of Lake Washington Boulevard and home to the city's largest remaining stand of tall trees. As the president of a native plants society argued, Seward Park was a prime example of "virgin forest, shrubs and flowers, growing in their native habitat," but thanks to poor maintenance, its "natural charm and beauty [had] been lost."[71] Public pressure by community clubs eventually forced the Parks Department to curtail its welfare program and abandon it by decade's end.

Even as some residents and city officials sought to regulate visitors' behavior in city parks, problems with urban wildlife confounded their efforts.

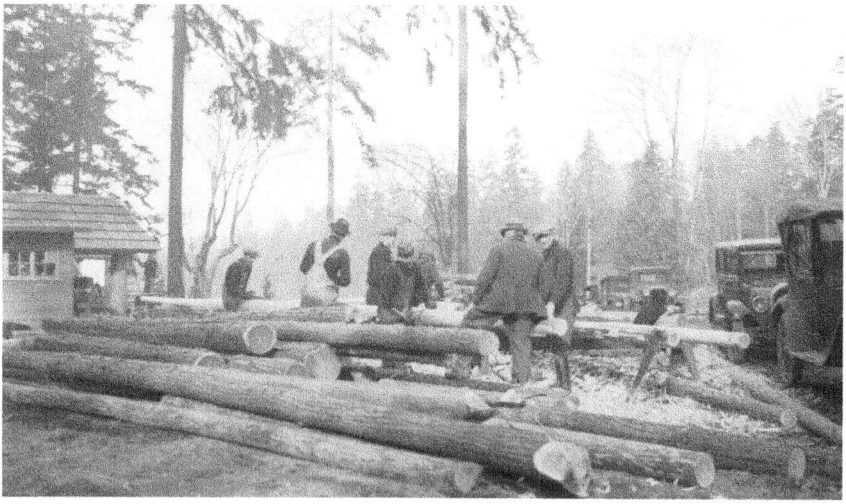

Figure 6. Works Progress Administration logging crew, Seward Park, 1936. Seattle Municipal Archives, Photograph Collection, Item 30316.

Since the 1910s, park officials encouraged the feeding of songbirds, squirrels, and waterfowl because bringing wildlife out into the open enhanced the qualities visitors wanted from their park experience. Feeding wildlife soon took on added urgency as habitat destruction, illegal hunting, and predation by domestic animals drove greater and greater numbers of wildlife into city parks. By 1936, park wardens were annually dispensing almost a ton and a half of seed in Woodland Park alone.[72] Creating room for animal refugees produced another set of problems by attracting unwanted pests, such as crows, or attractive species, such as geese and ducks, in such numbers that they became a nuisance. Canada geese at Green Lake Park soiled swimming beaches, while at Seward Park, marauding ducks grazed on residents' flowers and shrubs, but protests from the Audubon Society tied the hands of the Parks Department from culling waterfowl.[73]

Disgust over despoiled parks emphasized how Seattle's natural playground had lost some of its charms by the Depression. Physical changes intended to create spaces for recreation had instead yielded combat zones. Middle-class residents wanted environments wholly dedicated to leisure, devoid of production for food or commerce. Working-class residents did not see production and leisure, consumption and labor as separated because, in many instances, the landscapes where they worked were also the places where they played. Fights over who could claim these amenities and resources unfolded spatially. In some cases, what resulted was not the classic "tragedy of the commons" but a "tragedy of the commoners."[74] Excluded parties were not without recourse, but their reactions complicated the dilemmas that awaited environmental-minded consumers in the decades ahead.

Conclusion: The Nature and Culture of Fair Play

Historians have started to analyze how the rise of what became environmentalism in the postwar era grew in response to the earlier rise of modern consumerism. A spatial history of consumption can shed further light on the missing years before World War II because what happened in Seattle was not an isolated phenomenon. Squatters in San Francisco and New York City were pushed aside to build city parks in the late nineteenth and early twentieth centuries, and working-class residents in Hamilton and greater Toronto were expelled to make way for bourgeois bathing beaches.[75] Electrical utilities in turn-of-the-century Vancouver worked hand in glove with city officials to "to emancipate, entertain, and comfort new middle-class consumers" with cheap power at the expense of rural residents who suffered dammed rivers and drowned fields.[76] Real estate developers in interwar Los Angeles redrew park plans to put greenswards closest to the choicest new subdivisions, championing what would later be called sprawl as an environmental solution for wealthy urbanites yearning for the outdoors.[77] When Seattle's experiences are added to this list, an even broader perspective emerges.

At first glance, it may seem that when affluent Seattleites embraced outdoor recreation, they were embracing unproductive and pristine spaces of an ideal nature while rejecting the unsightly landscapes of industrial and commercial production. In strictly Marxian terms, recreational users suffered from a false consciousness because they were alienated from the real, legitimate means of production. This explanation is too easy because it suggests that the values of outdoor devotees were not interesting or legitimate in their own right. It also deflects attention from the complexity of their activities. Sport anglers and commercial fishermen, socialist campers and bourgeois mountaineers, picnickers and poachers were engaging in both production and consumption. One side deployed the cultural power of leisure by producing particular spaces and cultivating particular behaviors to promote outdoor play. The other side deployed the cultural power of labor to delimit specific locales where they could literally consume nature to advance producers' rights. At first, the two groups sometimes found common cause, but as each side sought to consolidate its gains, the social relations they espoused unleashed unexpected environmental changes that rebounded to their benefit or detriment. Neither side rejected capitalism. Instead, they breathed new life into its contradictions, splitting its meanings through divergent "aesthetic environmental ideologies."[78]

The story in this essay focuses on contests over outdoor recreation, but there are other stories to tell, stories about electricity and food, clean water and air, housing and open space, or other amenities that became as central to modern urban life as leisure. The allocation of these environmental benefits across the changing urban landscape is also a spatial story of consumption, one that ties directly into an implicit theme in many urban histories: environmental justice. The dynamics of consumption narrowed contests to fights between antagonistic consumers, or between consumers and producers. Social inequalities framed these battles and exposed the dream of the outdoor playground for what it was: a discriminatory way of defining the city and distributing its benefits.

The connections between consumer privilege and environmental protection have only intensified in the late twentieth century because the ideology of improving nature reached into Americans' pocketbooks and psyches decades before. Witness the fireworks between the so-called "New West" of urban consumers and the "Old West" of extractive industries, or rural timber workers and summer weekend vacationers in Maine's North Woods, to see how these conflicts play out in the present.[79] Historians need to rethink the origins of environmentalism and consumerism together, and one place to begin is in the city, where the ravenous quest for playing in nature got its start.

NOTES

Thanks to Connie Chiang, Andrew Isenberg, Kevin Kruse, Kathy Morse, Bruce Stadfeld, and Jay Taylor for their comments and suggestions, plus the participants and organizers of the "Nature of Cities" symposium at Princeton's Shelby Cullom Davis Center for Historical Studies. Special thanks to Amir Sheikh, who designed the custom maps, and to the Bowdoin College Faculty Research Fund, which helped me to acquire the images for this essay.

1. Caroline Sheldon, "Puget Sound Country and Alaska," *Chautauquan* 51 (July 1908): 175–77; also quoted in Janet Northam Russell and Jack W. Berryman, "Parks, Boulevards, and Outdoor Recreation: The Promotion of Seattle as an Ideal Residential City and Summer Resort, 1890–1910," *Journal of the West* 26 (January 1987): 9–10.

2. For a summary of this literature, see Lizabeth Cohen, "Is There an Urban History of Consumption?" *Journal of Urban History* 29 (January 2003): 87–106.

3. For the changing roles of nature and consumption, see Susan G. Davis, *Spectacular Nature: Corporate Culture and the Sea World Experience* (Berkeley: University of California Press, 1997); Jennifer Price, *Flight Maps: Adventures with Nature in Modern America* (New York: Basic Books, 1999); Matthew W. Klingle, "Spaces of Consumption in Environmental History," *History and Theory* 42 (December 2003): 94–110.

4. Western North American historians have produced several provocative studies that connect recreation and consumption through tourism, but few take into account the urban dimension. For salient examples, see Hal Rothman, *Devil's Bargains: Tourism in the Twentieth-Century American West* (Lawrence: University Press of Kansas, 1998); Bonnie Christensen, *Red Lodge and the Mythic West: Coal Miners to Cowboys* (Lawrence:

University Press of Kansas, 2002); William Peter Philpott, "Consuming Colorado: Landscapes, Leisure, and the Tourist Way of Life" (Ph.D. diss., University of Wisconsin, 2002); Connie Y. Chiang, "Monterey-by-the-Smell: Odors and Social Conflict on the California Coastline," *Pacific Historical Review* 73 (May 2004): 183–214, and "Novel Tourism: Nature, Industry, and Literature on Monterey's Cannery Row," *Western Historical Quarterly* 25 (Autumn 2004): 309–29; Annie Gilbert Coleman, *Ski Style: Sport and Culture in the Rockies* (Lawrence: University Press of Kansas, 2004). For a partial survey of this rich literature, see Joseph E. Taylor III, "The Many Lives of the New West," *Western Historical Quarterly* 25 (Summer 2004): 141–65.

5. Roy Rosenzweig, *Eight Hours for What We Will: Workers and Leisure in an Industrial City, 1870–1920* (New York: Cambridge University Press, 1983); Kathy Peiss, *Cheap Amusements: Working Women and Leisure in Turn-of-the-Century New York* (Philadelphia: Temple University Press, 1986); Lizabeth Cohen, *Making a New Deal: Industrial Workers in Chicago, 1919–1939* (New York: Cambridge University Press, 1990), and *A Consumer's Republic: The Politics of Mass Consumption in Postwar America* (New York: Knopf, 2003), pp. 193–289. While I use the term "North American" to include cities in Canada as well as the United States, I do not want to simplify the historical differences between the two nations in the name of inclusion. Joy Parr reminds us that in contrast to the United States, the Canadian federal government and a majority of Canadian citizens were willing "to accept continuing controls and persistent scarcity" well into the postwar period in exchange for greater social welfare. As Parr rightly notes, "to assume that all postwar consumer societies were the same, except in so far as their per capita income differed from that of the United States, is not a simplification but a disabling distortion." Parr's analysis of postwar Canadian consumer culture and politics is not entirely at odds with Cohen's thesis, but it is distinctive enough to be mentioned here. See *Domestic Goods: The Material, the Moral, and the Economic in the Postwar Years* (Toronto: University of Toronto Press, 1999), pp. 11, 32.

6. For examples, see Louis S. Warren, *The Hunter's Game: Poachers and Conservationists in Twentieth-Century America* (New Haven, Conn.: Yale University Press, 1997); Mark David Spence, *Dispossessing the Wilderness: Indian Removal and the Making of the National Parks* (New York: Oxford University Press, 1999); Karl Jacoby, *Crimes against Nature: Squatters, Poachers, Thieves, and the Hidden History of American Conservation* (Berkeley: University of California Press, 2001).

7. Andrew Hurley, *Environmental Inequalities: Class, Race, and Industrial Pollution in Gary, Indiana, 1945–1980* (Chapel Hill: University of North Carolina Press, 1995); and Adam Rome, *The Bulldozer in the Countryside: Suburban Sprawl and the Rise of American Environmentalism* (New York: Cambridge University Press, 2001). The standard survey of postwar environmentalism remains Samuel P. Hays, *Beauty, Health, and Permanence: Environmental Politics in the United States, 1955–1985* (New York: Cambridge University Press, 1987).

8. Kendrick A. Clements, *Hoover, Conservation, and Consumerism: Engineering the Good Life* (Lawrence: University Press of Kansas, 2000); and Paul S. Sutter, *Driven Wild: How the Fight against Automobiles Launched the Modern Wilderness Movement* (Seattle: University of Washington Press, 2002). See also David Louter, "Glaciers and Gasoline: The Making of a Windshield Wilderness, 1900–1915," in *Seen and Being Seen: Tourism in the American West*, ed. David M. Wrobel and Patrick T. Long

(Lawrence: University Press of Kansas, 2001), pp. 248–70; James Morton Turner, "From Woodcraft to 'Leave No Trace': Wilderness, Consumerism, and Environmentalism in Twentieth-Century America," *Environmental History* 7 (July 2002): 462–84.

9. The germinal work in this school of geography is Henri Lefebvre, *The Production of Space,* trans. Donald Nicholson-Smith (Cambridge, Mass.: Blackwell, 1991). Other geographers who have extended Lefebvre's ideas include Neil Smith, *Uneven Development: Nature, Capital, and the Production of Space* (Cambridge, Mass.: Blackwell, 1984, 1990); Edward W. Soja, *Postmodern Geographies: The Reassertion of Space in Critical Theory* (London: Verso, 1989); Mark Gottdiener, *The Social Production of Urban Space* (Austin: University of Texas Press, 1985); Allan Pred, *Making Histories and Constructing Human Geographies: The Social Transformation of Practice, Power Relations, and Consciousness* (Boulder, Colo.: Westview Press, 1990); and David Harvey, *Justice, Nature, and the Geography of Difference* (Cambridge, Mass.: Blackwell, 1996).

10. Henri Lefebvre, "The Right to the City," in *Writing on Cities,* trans. and ed. Eleonore Kofman and Elizabeth Lebas (Cambridge, Mass.: Blackwell, 1996), pp. 157–59; emphasis in the original.

11. Richard White, *"It's Your Misfortune and None of My Own": A New History of the American West* (Norman: University of Oklahoma Press, 1991), pp. 255–57; and Kathryn Morse, *The Nature of Gold: An Environmental History of the Klondike Gold Rush* (Seattle: University of Washington Press, 2003), pp. 40–88, 138–90.

12. Michael Chrzastowski, *Historical Changes to Lake Washington and the Route of the Lake Washington Ship Canal, King County, Washington* (Reston, Va.: United States Geological Survey, 1983); and George Blomberg, Charles Simenstad, and Paul Hickey, "Changes in Duwamish River Estuary Habitat Over the Past 125 Years," *Proceedings: First Annual Meeting on Puget Sound Research,* vol. 2 (Seattle: Puget Sound Water Quality Authority, 1988), pp. 437–54.

13. Arthur H. Dimock, "Preparing the Groundwork for a City: The Regrading of Seattle, Washington," *Transactions of the American Society of Civil Engineers* 92 (1928): 460–540; and Myra L. Phelps, *Public Works in Seattle: A Narrative History of the Engineering Department, 1875–1975* (Seattle: Department of Engineering, 1975), pp. 15–33.

14. Padraic Burke, "The City Beautiful Movement in Seattle" (M.A. thesis, University of Washington, 1973); William H. Wilson, *The City Beautiful Movement* (Baltimore: Johns Hopkins University Press, 1989), pp. 148–53.

15. *The City of Seattle, The County of King, The State of Washington* (Seattle: Chamber of Commerce, 1898), p. 15, Special Collections, University of Washington Libraries (hereafter UWL-SC).

16. Theodore Catton, *Wonderland: An Administrative History of Mount Rainier National Park* (Seattle: National Park Service, Cultural Resources Program, 1996), pp. 71–72.

17. Clarence B. Bagley, *History of Seattle from the Earliest Settlement to the Present Time* (Chicago; S. J. Clarke Publishing, 1916), pp. 523–29; George A. Frykman, "The Alaska-Yukon-Pacific Exposition, 1909," *Pacific Northwest Quarterly* 53 (July 1962): 89–99. On world's fairs as cultural markers of popular environmental perception or consumer culture, see Warren I. Susman, "The People's Fair: Cultural Contradictions of a Consumer Society," in *Culture as History: The Transformation of American Society in the Twentieth Century,* rev. ed. (New York: Oxford University Press, 1984), pp. 211–29; Neil Harris, "Museums, Merchandising, and Popular

Taste: The Struggle for Influence," and "Great American Fairs and American Cities: The Role of Chicago's Columbian Exposition," in *Cultural Excursions: Marketing Appetites and Cultural Tastes in Modern America* (Chicago: University of Chicago Press, 1990), pp. 56–81, 111–31. For the role of boosters in creating the modern West, see David M. Wrobel, *Promised Lands: Promotion, Memory, and the Creation of the American West* (Lawrence: University Press of Kansas, 2002).

18. Welford Beaton, *The City that Made Itself: A Literary and Pictorial Record of the Building of Seattle* (Seattle: Terminal Publishing Company, 1914), p. 69, UWL-SC.

19. *Wonderland '96* (St. Paul: Northern Pacific Railway, 1896); *Wonderland '97, A Story of the Northwest* (St. Paul: Northern Pacific Railway, 1897); *Wonderland '98* (St. Paul: Northern Pacific Railway, 1898); *Wonderland '99* (St. Paul: Northern Pacific Railway, 1899), UWL-SC. I take the term "mental territories" from Katherine G. Morrissey, *Mental Territories: Mapping the Inland Empire* (Ithaca, N.Y.: Cornell University Press, 1997).

20. For promoting Alaska, see e.g. "Alaska: Our Frontier Wonderland" (promotional literature, c. 1918), box 142, folders 2 and 5, Miles C. Poindexter Papers, UWL-SC.

21. *Seattle and King County: Statement of Facts Showing the Resources, Business Conditions and Progress of the Chief City and Largest County in the State of Washington* (Seattle: Chamber of Commerce, 1905), pp. 27–28, UWL-SC.

22. *Seattle Mail and Herald,* 26 August 1905.

23. For Boston and New York City, see Davis Strauss, "Toward a Consumer Culture: 'Adirondack Murray' and the Wilderness Vacation," *American Quarterly* 39 (Summer 1987): 270–86; Dona Brown, *Inventing New England: Regional Tourism in the Nineteenth Century* (Washington, D.C.: Smithsonian Institution Press, 1995); Richard Judd, *Common Lands, Common People: The Origins of Conservation in Northern New England* (Cambridge, Mass.: Harvard University Press, 1997), pp. 197–228; Philip G. Terrie, *Contested Terrain: A New History of Nature and People in the Adirondacks* (Syracuse, N.Y.: Syracuse University Press/The Adirondack Museum, 1997), pp. 44–82.

24. Quotation from *The American Wonderland: The Pacific Northwest* (Chicago, Burlington and Quincy RR, Northern Pacific Railway, Great Northern Railway, c. 1920), p. 3, box 28, Louis W. Hill Papers, James J. Hill Library, St. Paul; emphasis in original. For "Charmed Land" and "Evergreen Playground," see *Seattle: Metropolis of the Charmed Land of the American Continent, the Pacific Northwest* (Seattle: Chamber of Commerce, 1925?); *The Evergreen Playground in the Charmed Land: Seattle, Center of a Scenic Wonderland* (Seattle: Chamber of Commerce, 1929?), UWL-SC. For the "See America First" movement, refer to Marguerite S. Shaffer, *See America First: Tourism and National Identity, 1880–1940* (Washington, D.C.: Smithsonian Institute Press, 2001).

25. *The American Wonderland,* pp. 19–20. For the urban dimensions of tourism in the early twentieth century, see Earl Pomeroy, *In Search of the Golden West: The Tourist in Western* America (New York: Knopf, 1957); Catherine Cocks, *Doing the Town: The Rise of Urban Tourism in the United States, 1850–1915* (Berkeley: University of California Press, 2001); J. Mark Souther, "Landscapes of Leisure: Building an Urban History of Tourism," *Journal of Urban History* 30 (January 2004): 257–65.

26. "The Spirit of Play," *Welfare* 1 (November 1913): 8–9, UWL-SC. For therapeutic leisure and the rise of vacations, see T. J. Jackson Lears, *No Place of Grace:*

Antimodernism and the Transformation of American Culture, 1880–1920 (New York: Pantheon Books, 1981); Cindy S. Aron, *Working at Play: A History of Vacations in the United States* (New York: Oxford University Press, 1999).

27. Almira Bailey, "The Charmed Land," in *Seattle and the Charmed Land* (Seattle: Chamber of Commerce, 1930?), p. 2. UWL-SC. For promotion of outdoor sports, see *Seattle Mail and Herald,* 16 November 1901 and 16 April 1902; *Seattle Argus,* 28 March 1896 and 18 December 1897; *Seattle Post-Intelligencer,* 11 May 1898 and 1 June 1902; Virginia Miller, "The Development of Leisure Time Activities in Seattle" (M.A. thesis, University of Washington, 1980), pp. 183–86.

28. *Brief History of the Washington State Good Roads Association* (Seattle: Washington State Good Roads Association, 1939), UWL-SC; Norman Hayner, "Auto Camps in the Evergreen Playground," *Social Forces* 9 (December 1930): 256–66.

29. Peter J. Schmitt, *Back to Nature: The Arcadian Myth in Urban America* (New York: Oxford University Press, 1969), pp. 20–32.

30. Quotations from *Seattle Mail and Herald,* 19 December 1903 and 13 January 1906.

31. Quotation from *Seattle Post-Intelligencer,* 18 July 1909. For the history of the Mountaineers, see Jim Kjeldsen, *The Mountaineers: A History* (Seattle: The Mountaineers, 1998); George A. Frykman, *Seattle's Historian and Promoter: The Life of Edmond Stephen Meany* (Pullman: Washington State University Press, 1998), pp. 27–126. For histories of the Mazamas and the Sierra Club, see *Mazama History* (Portland, Ore.: The Mazamas, 1932); Michael P. Cohen, *The History of the Sierra Club, 1892–1970* (San Francisco: Sierra Club Press, 1988); and Erik L. Weiselberg, "Ascendancy of the Mazamas: Environment, Identity, and Mountain Climbing in Oregon, 1870 to 1930" (Ph.D. diss., University of Oregon, 1999).

32. *The Mountaineer* 1 (1907): 45–48, and 2 (1909): 4–12, UWL-SC. For descriptions of the required "personal outfit" for one annual trip to Mount Rainer, see *Mountaineer Bulletin* 2 (June 1912): 2, UWL-SC.

33. J. N. Bowman, "Local Walks: Seattle Local Walks," *The Mountaineer* 8 (1915): 78; see also Edmond S. Meany, "Objects of Our Club," ibid., 3 (1910): 6–7, 70–72, UWL-SC.

34. Anna Louise Strong, "Plans made by Camp Seattle for Camps on Rainier, 1917," box 9, folder 10, Anna Louise Strong Papers, UWL-SC.

35. *Co-Operative Campers Bulletin* (Seattle, 1923–24), UWL-SC.

36. Charles P. LeWarne, *Utopias on Puget Sound, 1885–1915* (Seattle: University of Washington Press, 1975); Dana Frank, *Purchasing Power: Consumer Organizing, Gender, and the Seattle Labor Movement, 1919–1929* (New York: Cambridge University Press, 1994), pp. 40–65, 108–38, 212–46.

37. Anna Louise Strong to Sydney Strong, c. 1916, box 3, folder 9a, Anna Louise Strong Papers; Strong, *I Change Worlds: The Remaking of an American* (New York: Garden City Publishing, 1937), p. 57.

38. Stephanie Francine Ogle, "Anna Louise Strong: Progressive and Propagandist" (Ph.D. diss., University of Washington, 1981), pp. 112–200; Catton, *Wonderland,* pp. 260–73.

39. Lloyd Anderson, "The Beginning of Recreational Equipment Cooperative," 22 October 1976; "The Beginning of the Climbing Course," 10 February 1968; "The Cooperative Group," c. 1938; Anderson to Ed Kennedy, 11 October 1939;

Roffe Bedayan to Anderson, 16 November 1941; Climbers' Notebook, 1937–1940; all box 1, Lloyd Anderson Papers, UWL-SC. For the history of REI, see Harvey Manning, *REI: Fifty Years of Climbing Together: The REI Story* (Seattle: Recreational Equipment Cooperative, Inc., 1988).

40. Robert S. Lynd and Helen Merrill Lynd, *Middletown: A Study in American Culture* (New York: Harcourt, Brace, 1929), pp. 225–314.

41. Robert Spector, *The Legend of Eddie Bauer* (Lyme, Conn.: Greenwich Publishing Group, 1994), pp. 9–41.

42. Schmitt, *Back to Nature*, p. 79.

43. Frank B. Cooper to Board of Directors, Seattle School District, 7 April 1915, box 2, folder: School Gardens, 1915–1919, Superintendent's Files, Seattle School District Archives and Records Center; see also *Thirty-fourth Annual Report of the Public Schools, Seattle, Washington* (Quinquennial Report: 1916–21), pp. 75–78, Annual Reports, Seattle School District Archives and Records Center.

44. Lou Evans, "A City Teaches Swimming," and Ben Evans, "Seattle's 43 Playfields, 10 Beaches and 39 Parks Provide Complete Program," *Western City* 7 (May 1931): 26–28. *Nineteenth Annual Report, Seattle Board of Park Commissioners* (1922), pp. 21–22; *Report of the Department of Parks, City of Seattle, 1923–1930*, pp. 112–13, 118–21, and 123–24, box 3, folder 7 and box 4, folder 4, Don Sherwood Parks History Collection (hereafter DSPHC), Seattle Parks and Recreation Department, Seattle Municipal Archives; Vern Allen Armstrong, "The First Fifty Years of Municipal Recreation Programs in the State of Washington" (M.A. thesis, University of Washington, 1956), pp. 49–92.

45. Herbert Hoover to Charles D. Walcott, 26 February 1924, box 272, folder: Hoover, Herbert—Memberships, National, F–P, Herbert Hoover Papers, Hoover Presidential Library, as quoted in Clements, *Hoover, Conservation, and Consumerism*, p. 90.

46. *Nineteenth Annual Report, Seattle Board of Park Commissioners* (1922). p. 20, box 3, folder 7, DSPHC.

47. Clark E. Schurman, "Monitor Rock," *The Mountaineer*, 15 December 1938, p. 20. William G. Long, Remarks at Dedication of Youth Camp, 8 November 1941, "Story Behind Camp Long and Schurman Rock," c. 1941, "Camp Long Day Camp," c. 1941, box 3, folders 15, 16; Ben Evans, Address to Winter Sports Symposium, National Recreation Association Conference, 13–15 April 1938, and "Snoqualmie Ski Bowl Frolic and Hike," 22 August 1939, box 23, folder 14; all Ben Evans Recreation Program Collection, Seattle Parks and Recreation Department, Seattle Municipal Archives.

48. Edmond S. Meany, "The Coming City of Puget Sound," 24 June 1929, box 59, folder 4, Edmond S. Meany Papers, UWL-SC; see also *Annual Report, Seattle Board of Park Commissioners* (1928); *Survey of Recreation Facilities, Parks Department and School District No. 1* (1928); and "Comparison of the Present Park System and the Proposed Metropolitan Park District System," c. 1929, box 3, folder 21–23 and box 4, folder 2, DSPHC.

49. Hiram M. Chittenden, "Sentiment versus Utility in the Treatment of National Scenery," *Pacific Monthly* 23 (January 1910): 37–38.

50. Paul Whitham, "Seattle Prepares for Great Motor Fleet," *Pacific Motor Boat* 2 (November 1911): 12.

51. Howard Droker, *Seattle's Unsinkable Houseboats: An Illustrated History* (Seattle: Watermark Press, 1977), pp. 33–41, 49–62; John Herbert Geoghegan, "The Migratory Worker in Seattle: A Study in Social Disorganization and Exploitation" (M.A. thesis, University of Washington, 1923), pp. 35–91; and Gordon Beebe, "Ecological Aspects of Substandard Housing in Seattle" (M.A. thesis, University of Washington, 1939), pp. 44–49.

52. Quotations from *Seattle Post-Intelligencer*, 2 August 1908.

53. Barton Warren Evermann and Seth Eugene Meek, "A Report upon Salmon Investigations in the Columbia River and Elsewhere on the Pacific Coast in 1896," *Bulletin of the United States Fish Commission for 1897* (Washington, D.C.: Government Printing Office), pp. 34–47; R. Rathbun, "A Review of the Fisheries in the Contiguous Waters of the State of Washington and British Columbia," *Report of the United States Fish Commission for the Year Ending June 30, 1899* (Washington, D.C.: Government Printing Office, 1890): pp. 251–350. For commercial fishing on the Duwamish, see L. H. Darwin, State Fish Commissioner, to Governor Louis F. Hart, 1 October 1919, box 2J-1-18, Fisheries Commission File, 1919, Governors' Papers, Governor Louis F. Hart Group (hereafter Hart Group), Washington State Archives.

54. Matthew W. Klingle, "Fluid Dynamics: Water, Power, and the Reengineering of Seattle's Duwamish River," *Journal of the West* 44 (Summer 2005), forthcoming. For details on salmon runs, see Jonathan L. Reisland, Commissioner and Game Warden, *Sixteenth and Seventeenth Annual Reports of the State Fish Commissioner and Game Warden, 1905–1906* (Olympia, Wash.: C. W. Corham, 1907), pp. 15–16. For further complaints about pollution and stream blockages, see the following Washington State Department of Fisheries (hereafter WSDF) Annual Reports: *First Annual* (1890), pp. 25–30; *Ninth Annual* (1898), p. 6; *Tenth/Eleventh Annual* (1899–1900), pp. 16–18; *Twenty-Second/Twenty-Third* (1911–12), pp. 95–104; *Twenty-Fourth/Twenty-Fifth* (1913–15), pp. 27–28.

55. W. T. Isted, Secretary, Northwestern Tow Boats Owners' Association, to L. H. Darwin, State Fish Commissioner, 19 December 1919, box 2J-1-18, Fisheries Commission File, 1919, Hart Group.

56. For class interests and salmon politics, see Joseph E. Taylor III, *Making Salmon: An Environmental History of the Northwest Fisheries Crisis* (Seattle: University of Washington Press, 1999), pp. 166–202.

57. L. H. Darwin, State Fish Commissioner, *Twenty-Eighth and Twenty-Ninth Annual Reports of the State Fish Commissioner, 1917–1919* (Olympia, Wash.: State Printer, 1919), pp. 10–13. Arthur McEvoy also details how state power was deployed against immigrant fisheries in California in the late nineteenth century in efforts to regulate declining stocks; see Arthur F. McEvoy, *The Fisherman's Problem: Ecology and Law in the California Fisheries, 1850–1980* (New York: Cambridge University Press, 1986), pp. 65–119.

58. Petitions to Governor Louis F. Hart, 5 January 1920, box 2J-1-18, Fisheries Commission File, 1920, Hart Group.

59. Quotation from Frank L. Jackson to Governor Louis F. Hart, 13 February 1920, Box 2J-1-18, Fisheries Commission File, 1919, Hart Group. For closing the Duwamish River and Shilshole Bay, see "Notice of Closing of Stream to Fishing," (3 February 1920—draft), box 2J-1-18, Fisheries Commission File, 1919, Hart Group; "Before the State Fisheries Board," Order No. 18 (1921), box 2, Hearings of State

Fisheries Board, vol. H7, Department of Fisheries, Administration Library, Acc. 74-12-1115, WSDF; "Test of Duwamish Closing," *Pacific Fisherman* 18 (February 1920): 30. For responses by sportsmen and industrialists, see e.g. Petition, 17 April 1922, box 3, Correspondence of State Fisheries Board, vol. L5, Department of Fisheries, Administration Library, Acc. 74-12-1115, WSDF. This last petition included a letter of thanks signed by seventy-three sportsmen and commercial fishers, including several Japanese and Scandinavian commercial operators, who opposed unregulated net fishing by aliens and Indians.

60. Quotations from W. C. Sanford, A. Stass, and William Russell ["Committee"], to Hon. Louis F. Hart, 28 November 1919, box 2J-1-18, Fisheries Commission File, 1919, Hart Group; and "Statement of R. Q. Hall, Hearing on Puget Sound Fishery Matters," 20 June 1921, box 2, Hearings of State Fisheries Board, vol. H1, Department of Fisheries, Administration Library, Acc. 74-12-1115, WSDF.

61. For arrest records, see *Annual Reports of the State Fish Commissioner: Twenty-Eighth and Twenty-Ninth* (1917–19), p. 162; *Thirtieth and Thirty-First* (1919–21), pp. 202, 293–94; *Thirty-Second and Thirty-Third* (1921–23), pp. 44–45, 104; *Thirty-Fourth and Thirty-Fifth* (1923–25), pp. 63–64, 128; *Thirty-Sixth and Thirty-Seventh* (1925–27), pp. 123–24, 203. The Department of Fisheries and Game stopped printing detailed arrest records following the 1925–27 biennium. See also *Seattle Times,* 1, 6, 11 October 1928. For environmental banditry, see Jacoby, *Crimes Against Nature,* pp. 1–6.

62. *Seattle Times,* 31 July 1928, 18 August 1929; H. L. Dillaway, "Trout Fishing," *Northwest Sportsman* 1 (April 1932): 2–4, 7.

63. For details on the Seward Park hatchery, see *Annual Report, Board of Park Commissioners* (1934), p. 15. "Lake Washington Fish Ponds," c. 1934, box 5, folder 2; and A. M. Young, District #2 Engineer, Washington Emergency Relief Administration, to W. J. Dahl, 31 August 1934, box 43, folder 12; both DSPHC. For details of the Issaquah hatchery, see L. A. Royal and Allen Seymour, "Building New Salmon Runs," *Progressive Fish Culturist* 52 (1940). The sockeye planted in Lake Washington were evolutionarily distinct from the indigenous kokanee or land-locked sockeye; see *Twenty-Eighth and Twenty-Ninth Annual Reports of the State Fish Commissioner, 1917–1919,* p. 89; Andrew Paul Hendry, "Sockeye Salmon (*Onchorhynchus nerka*) in Lake Washington: An Investigation of Ancestral Origins, Population Differentiation and Local Adaptation" (Ph.D. diss., University of Washington, 1995), pp. 1–13, 135–39.

64. For dams and salmon, see Director of Fisheries and Director of Game to H. D. Towler, Superintendent, Water Department, 27 February 1936; B. M. Brennan, Director, Department of Fisheries, to W. C. Morse, Superintendent, Seattle Water Department, 1 September 939; and Morse to Brennan, 12 September 1939; all Cedar River Watershed Collection, Cedar River Watershed Education Center Library, Seattle Public Utilities. For a later incident of recreational and industrial conflicts over fishing, see Kristin M. Szylvian, "Transforming Lake Michigan into the 'World's Greatest Fishing Hole': The Environmental Politics of Lake Michigan's Great Lakes Sports Fishing, 1965–1985," *Environmental History* 9 (January 2004): 102–27.

65. Seattle Audubon Society to Game Commission for King County, 10 January 1924, box 1, folder 12, Seattle Audubon Society Records (hereafter SASR), UWL-SC; see also May J. Compton, President, Seattle Audubon Society, to Board of Park Commissioners, 24 November 1919, box 2, folder 24, DSPHC.

66. Seattle Audubon Society to Game Commission for King County, 10 January 1924, box 1, folder 12, SASR; see also May J. Compton, President, Seattle Audubon Society, to Board of Park Commissioners, 24 November 1919, box 2, folder 24, DSPHC. For Audubon outings in and around Seattle prior to World War II, see "Field Trip Reports," box 14, folders 11–12, SASR.

67. Ella B. Rowntree to Mrs. H. F. Alexander, 15 October 1928, box 39, folder 10; Sigrid M. Frisch to E. R. Hoffman, Engineer, Seattle Parks Department, 9 March 1930, box 41, folder 2; both DSPHC.

68. A. S. Kerry to City Council and Park Board, 2 July 1937, box 46, folder 17, DSPHC. For the closing of the camp, see *Report of the Department of Parks, City of Seattle, 1923–1930*, 47–48, box 4, folder 4, DSPHC.

69. Kerry to various recipients and Board of Park Commissioners to all Community Clubs, 29 September 1928, box 3, folder 22, DSPHC. Paul Sutter argues that cars and parks were seen as irreconcilable by the end of the 1930s; see *Driven Wild*, pp. 4–6, 100–111, and passim. But not all scholars agree that nature and parks were incompatible in the pre–World War II era; see David Louter, "Windshield Wilderness: The Automobile and the Meaning of National Parks in Washington State," (Ph.D. diss., University of Washington, 2000).

70. Quotation from *Annual Report, Board of Park Commissioners* (1934), p. 12, boxes 22–23; for unemployed welfare programs, see *Fifth Annual Report of the Board of Park Commissioners* (1907–8), pp. 22–23, box 4, folder 4; *Report of the Department of Parks, City of Seattle, 1923–1930* (1931), pp. 48–49, box 5, folder 2; all DSPHC; Armstrong, "First Fifty Years of Municipal Recreation Programs," pp. 88–90.

71. Quotation from Mrs. Alexander F. McEwan, President, Washington State Society for the Conservation of Wildflowers and Native Trees, to Board of Park Commissioners, 1 April 1936, box 43, folder 13, DSPHC. For protests against unemployed laborers and relief camps, see e.g. "Petition to Board of Park Commissioners," 18 October 1934; Josiah Collins, Seattle Chamber of Commerce, to Board of Park Commissioners, 27 March 1936; George S. DeLappe, Chairman, Committee to Investigate Seward Park, to D. C. Conover, President, Consolidated South District Commercial Club, 9 April 1936, box 43, folder 13; and Erickson to F. F. Powell, 3 July 1936, box 23, folder 10 and box 5, folder 10, DSPHC; see also "Petition Against Logging in Seward Park," file 150912, Seattle City Clerk's Files, Seattle Municipal Archives.

72. *Annual Report of the Board of Park Commissioners* (1906–7), pp. 14–15, box 1/9; *Annual Report, Board of Park Commissioners* (1937), box 5, folder 11, DSPHC; Mrs. L. Houston Reusch, Bird Chairman, National Council of State Garden Clubs, *The Seattle Wren* 6 (April 1938): 1, 4; and "Bird Feeding in the Arboretum," ibid., 8 (April 1940): 4, box 12, folder 15, SASR. For the effects of songbird hunting, see P. F. Appel to Board of Park Commissioners, 18 September 1916, box 42, folder 1, DSPHC.

73. For feeding and pests, see *Annual Report, Board of Park Commissioners* (1938), box 5, folder 13, DSPHC. For crows, see W. M. Elliott to Simon Burnett, President, Seattle Park Board, 12 August 1929; *Annual Work Report, Parks and Boulevard Division, Seattle Parks Department* (1943); box 45, folder 22 and box 5, folder 17, DSPHC. For waterfowl problems, see Donna M. Henderson, Secretary, Lakewood Community Club, to Seattle Park Board, 14 November 1936; H. M. Read, Commissioner of

Health, to Board of Park Commissioners, 27 April and 9 May 1920, box 34, folder 21 and box 29, folder 1, DSPHC. For support of the Seward Park refuge, see "History of the Seattle Audubon Society" (c. 1955–56), pp. 9–10, 30, box 1, folder 1, SASR; *Seattle Post-Intelligencer,* 5 January 1939.

74. I take the term "tragedy of the commoners" from Bonnie J. McCay, "The Culture of the Commoners: Historical Observations of Old and New World Fisheries," in *The Question of the Commons: The Culture and Ecology of Communal Resources,* ed. Bonnie J. McCay and James M. Acheson (Tucson: University of Arizona Press, 1987), pp. 195–216.

75. Terrence Young, "Modern Urban Parks," *Geographical Review* 85 (October 1991): 535–51; Roy Rosenzweig and Elizabeth Blackmar, *The Park and Its People: A History of Central Park* (Ithaca, N.Y.: Cornell University Press, 1992), pp. 59–91; Ken Cruikshank and Nancy B. Bouchier, "'The Heritage of the People Closed Against Them': Class, Environment, and the Shaping of Burlington Beach, 1870s–1890s," *Urban History Review/Revue d'histoire urbaine* 30 (October 2001): 40–55, and "The War on the Squatters, 1920–1940: Hamilton's Boathouse Community and the Re-creation of Recreation on Burlington Bay," *Labour/Le Travail* 51 (Spring 2003): 9–46.

76. Bruce Stadfeld, "Electric Space: Social and Natural Transformations in British Columbia's Hydroelectric Industry to World War II" (Ph.D. diss., University of Manitoba, 2002), pp. 166–67.

77. Greg Hise and William Deverell, "Private Power, Public Space," in *Eden by Design: The 1930 Olmsted-Bartholomew Plan for the Los Angeles Region* (Berkeley: University of California Press, 2000), pp. 1–63.

78. Peter Walker, "Reconsidering 'Regional' Political Ecologies: Toward a Political Ecology of the Rural American West," *Progress in Human Geography* 27 (March 2003): 17.

79. Taylor, "The Many Lives of the New West," pp. 162–65; Richard W. Judd and Christopher W. Beach, *Natural States: The Environmental Imagination in Maine, Oregon, and the Nation* (Washington, D.C.: Resources for the Future, 2003), pp. 167–252; Hal Clifford, "The Gear Biz," *High Country News,* 27 October 2003.

Part III

Cities Deconstructed

8

The Palenque Paradox

Bush Cities, Bushmen, and the Bush

Emmanuel Kreike

The urban environment is often seen as the consummate cultural landscape, and as the polar opposite of pristine Nature or "wilderness." "Aboriginal" people such as, for example, the Bushmen or San are frequently seen as indicators of unspoiled wilderness while their lifestyles are seen as the antithesis to urban Western life.[1] But the wilderness expanses of Central America and Africa contain the ruins of a large number of "lost" cities, such as, for example, Palenque and Great Zimbabwe.[2] The Bushmen and their environments similarly may have not been as "wild" as has sometimes been presumed. At the same time that European travelers uncovered Palenque and Great Zimbabwe, the Bushmen/San of southwestern Africa displayed behavior that seemed in sharp contradiction to that expected of archetypical nomadic "Stone Age hunters and gatherers." Armed with the latest firearms technology, they engaged in commercial hunting, were involved in mining copper and iron, and lived in permanent villages. The reigning paradigm of environmental change is premised on a Nature-Culture dichotomy with a single pathway of linear change away from a state of (virgin) Nature. The presence of urban ruins in the jungles and plains of Central America and Africa, and the degree to which Bushmen society was in fact embedded in Culture rather than Nature, are problematic. At the very least, these facts constitute a paradox.[3]

Bush Cities and the Bush

The "jungles" or "bush" of Africa, Central America, and Southeast Asia are not only a treasure throve of biodiversity, but also home to some of the most impressive remnants of urban civilizations, including Great Zimbabwe in Zimbabwe, Palenque in Mexico, and Angkor Wat in Cambodia.[4] Evidence of the past presence of cultural landscapes in what at present is defended as the last relics of pristine Nature is paradoxical: how can the site of the historical city of Palenque be pristine Nature?

Two conceptions have somewhat eased the tension. One is the idea that premodern societies somehow "lived by Nature," i.e. sustained themselves within the bounds and limits of their natural environments. This idea is most explicitly expressed in the literature about Native Americans, the African Bushmen, and Pygmies and other "aboriginal" peoples.[5] But on the other hand, indigenous settled agricultural societies are sometimes seen as being environmentally destructive: theories about the decline of Central American urban societies, for example, attribute their demise to environmental overexploitation.[6]

The second conception is much more implicit. The remnants of urban vestiges in "wild" Africa and the "rainforests" of Central America are depicted as though they are entirely isolated from the surrounding natural ecosystems. The most dramatic image is the view that Palenque offers its visitors: the white stone of its buildings contrasts sharply with the towering green jungle that embraces it. It seems an anomaly, vulnerable even, its frailty punctuated by machete-wielding crews of men who seem to be engaged in an endless battle to keep the wilderness at bay. The human corruption of Nature thus seems confined, effectively quarantined. At least until recently, archaeological bias towards the spectacular and the monumental led to a disregard for the mundane, including details surrounding the daily functioning of residential sites and due appreciation for the size of the populations: by 1960 only the largest structures had been excavated.[7] Another factor that prejudiced against recognizing (sub)tropical urban societies as "urban" was their peculiar (that is, in comparison to the norm of urban societies in the temperate zones) climatic, geographical, and demographic traits. Precolonial urban centers in the (sub)tropics were often subject to a climate with a sharp dry season–rainy season variability. They also frequently were not located along a major (permanent) river, and settlement may have been less concentrated than in premodern Europe.[8]

In *Nature's Metropolis* William Cronon argues against the separation of urban and nonurban and human and natural worlds. He demonstrates that urban Chicago and its rural and wilderness hinterland were part of a continuum, and that they were mutually dependent upon one another. Chicago's urban growth led to a cutover of the forest regions to its north and transformed the bison prairies to its west into wheat fields and cattle range.[9] Although in perhaps less spectacular ways, African, Central American, and Southeast Asian urban centers were connected to and dependent on large hinterlands, leading to significant environmental change.[10] Precolonial urban centers were large and numerous. The Aztec capital of Tenochtitlán boasted 250,000 inhabitants, five times the population of contemporary London. Tikal in the eighth century was surrounded by expanses of suburbs. Nohmul's remains cover an area of thirty-five square kilometers. Precious little vacant land remained in the area immediately around the central pyramid group at Chunchumil because the site contained twenty-four hundred housing complexes with a total estimated population of twelve thousand on a mere six square kilometers. Mexico alone counts ten thousand known sites of Meso-American cities and towns and Guatemala has another fourteen hundred. Great Zimbabwe had a population of up to thirty thousand inhabitants and over fifty other sites with significant ruins are associated with it.[11]

Construction and maintenance of the urban structures and their populations must have been a severe drain on the hinterlands. The stone used to construct Angkor Wat came from quarries thirty kilometers away. Maintenance was costly: eighty thousand people in 3,140 villages were assigned to the upkeep of a single temple in Angkor Wat built by king Jayavarman VII in the twelfth century.[12] The Incas had a centralized system that supplied urban centers with firewood that originated from the Andean forests.[13]

Food production requirements to sustain the urban populations also support the concept of an urban-rural continuum. Intensive horticulture in garden plots that included fruit trees was found within the confines of Maya cities and towns.[14] Much of the food, however, must have originated from the rural areas. Before the late 1970s, pre-Columbian agriculture was thought to have been dominated by the *milpa,* temporary fields in a slash-and-burn cultivation system. Research in the 1970s and 1980s, however, found evidence of much more intensive forms of cultivation, based on raised fields and intricate systems of irrigation, and water harvesting and storage, suggesting dramatic levels of pre-Columbian Indian environmental manipulation.[15]

Recent revisionist scholarship has criticized the view that highly intensive land use largely dominated pre-Columbian environments. It argues that the evidence of intensive agriculture cannot simply be extrapolated from a limited number of cases. Instead, the literature proposes the concept of a mosaic, maintaining that the pre-Columbian Maya landscapes were marked by high differentiation in land use with areas of less intensively used land interspersed with pockets of intensive land use in a dispersed settlement pattern.[16] Fields were also not necessarily close to the main residences.[17] Minerals and forest products were acquired even beyond the agricultural hinterlands of the cities and towns. The Mayan upland forests, for example, were long considered to be of minor importance to the Maya, but Dunham points out that they were relatively close to urban centers. The upland forests 100–150 kilometers from Tikal were the source of many sought-after minerals and sizable settlements to extract forest resources were located wherever water was available.[18] In addition, urban centers and their hinterlands were connected to one another through intricate networks of exchange. This is as true for nineteenth- and twentieth-century Chicago as it was for Tikal, Palenque, and Great Zimbabwe. Great Zimbabwe traded as far southwest as Toranju near the Makgadigadi Pans in central Botswana, and as far north as

Ingombe Ilede in the Zambezi Valley, and it was a core area in the Indian Ocean trade system that stretched as far east as China.[19]

This suggests that much if not all of Meso-America may have been a domesticated environment. Indeed, the seemingly "pristine forests" of the Maya lowlands are less than four hundred years old and, moreover, are not identical to the pre-Mayan vegetation.[20] "Primordial" forest wilderness in Latin America such as that found at La Selva research station in Costa Rica revealed human use as evidenced by pre-Columbian sites with charcoal and ceramic remnants.[21] Many tropical forests are cultural rather than natural systems. Every forested landscape bears evidence of human interventions over the course of the millennia.[22]

This may be equally true for Africa, often considered the "wild" continent par excellence. Africa's game parks and nature preserves are rarely pristine. Most protected areas have long histories of human use. As anyone who has flown between Johannesburg and Maputo can attest, the southern Kruger Park is pockmarked by the remnants of human settlements. The northern Kruger Park was also inhabited during the early 1900s. When much of the South African Lowveld along the Mozambican border was transformed into what became the Kruger Park, some of the inhabitants were expelled while others were initially retained as gamekeepers and other staff. The Makuleke were forcibly expelled from the Parfuri Triangle in the far northern part of the park during the 1960s. Thus, although the first game warden of the Kruger Park propagandized the park as an African Eden, it was hardly pristine Nature.[23]

Wilderness in another remote corner of southern Africa was similarly not so "pristine." In the late 1800s, the Okalongo region in the middle Ovambo flood plain was described as an uninhabited hunters' paradise. Yet, when refugees from the northern Ovambo flood plain settled the area in the 1920s and 1930s, they encountered evidence of the presence of earlier settlement: fruit trees, water holes, water reservoirs, and pottery fragments. They attributed these relics of a past humanized landscape to the prosperous kingdom of Haudanu, which was abandoned after a destructive war in the early 1800s. By the 1960s, the refugees and their descendants had once more transformed the Okalongo wilderness into a thriving and densely settled village landscape.[24]

Whereas war and population dislocation led to the recolonization of the Okalongo wilderness, the same processes had an opposite effect just north of Okalongo on the Angolan side of the border with Namibia. By the 1990s, local inhabitants described large areas directly north of the Angolan-Namibian border on the western side of the Ovambo flood plain as wilderness.[25] Yet, less than a century earlier, the same areas were described as lush fruit tree–shaded expanses of adjoining farms and fields.[26] Indeed, tree species considered to be wild may be neither wild nor wilderness trees. As is the case with other African indigenous fruit trees as well as with various indigenous fruit trees in Latin America, marula trees (*Sclerocarya birrea*) in north-central Namibia are the result of and thus evidence of past human settlement and/or intensive past human use. Thus, they are indicators of culture in nature and not the other way around, i.e. a relic of (lost) nature in a cultural landscape.[27]

Indeed, the early twentieth-century northern Ovambo flood plain, which supported the Ombadja and Oukwanyama kingdoms, was amongst the most densely settled areas of what is modern Angola. The estimated population of pre–First World War Oukwanyama was from 60,000 to 120,000 and that of the smaller Ombadja kingdoms, located on the western side of the northern flood plain, may have been between 15,000 and 60,000 inhabitants. Northern flood plain villages often abutted one another.[28] The semi-arid environment could only sustain such large populations because its inhabitants had constructed a water harvesting and storage infrastructure that relied on shallow water holes or wells.[29]

Warfare, famine, and disease associated with colonial conquest, and heavy taxation and forced labor between 1900 and 1930, led to massive mortality and flight, decimating the northern flood plain populations and triggering the abandonment of entire villages and districts, especially in the southern parts of the Ombadja region. By the 1930s, many of the formerly most densely Ombadja districts were uninhabited and entirely overgrown by bush vegetation. One Portuguese source estimated that between 1915 and 1918 alone, the population density of Angola as a whole declined from nine persons per square kilometer to six persons. A Portuguese official report from 1919 claimed that the pre-1915 population density in Oukwanyama was eight persons per square kilometer and for the Ombadjas, twelve persons per square kilometer. The figures may have been inflated because they legitimized indemnity claims against Germany, but they nevertheless illustrate that the region was considered to be fairly densely settled. In the context of the descriptions of the kingdoms as expanses of farms, fields, and villages with an extensive water infrastructure, these reports emphasize the extent to which barely a century earlier, the 1990s wilderness had appeared to be very much like a semiurban environment, or, at the very least, a "managed mosaic" environment similar to that of "rural" lowland Central America.[30]

Bushmen and the Bush

Even the "last wildernesses" that are home to "Stone Age" hunter-gatherers, the Bushmen/San and Pygmies, are not true wilderness.[31] Bushman/San communities in the late nineteenth- and early twentieth-century border region in south-central Angola and north-central Namibia did not simply live by nature, but in fact significantly shaped their environment. As Wilmsen and Gordon have demonstrated, the "San" or 'Bushmen" of nineteenth- and twentieth-century Botswana and Namibia were not "wild," that is isolated, small-scale, subsistence, nomadic hunter-gatherer societies. Gordon, for example, documents that Namibian Bushmen controlled Tsumeb copper mining and engaged in commercial hunting.[32] Ovambo kings supplied ammunition and the most advanced firearms to their Bushmen business partners for elephant hunting, and the king and the hunter each received half of the ivory.[33] Qualifying the region's Bushmen as "Stone Age" subsistence hunter-gatherers seems untenable given the significant evidence that they were entrepreneurs involved in mining and in commercial elephant hunting in addition to hiring themselves out to Ovambo kings as bodyguards and executioners.[34]

Their environment similarly did not constitute "wilderness." The Bushmen/San who lived in or adjacent to the Ovambo flood plain because they were the main elephant hunters in the region may have significantly contributed to the demise of elephant herds in southern Angola and northern Namibia during the second half of the nineteenth century (and probably to the overhunting of other game).[35] The decimation of the region's elephant population in the late nineteenth century, which was hastened by the 1897 rinderpest epizootic, coincided with a dramatic decline in the fortunes of the region's San communities—another possible indicator of how dependent the San had become on the commercial hunt and the trade in game products. By the early twentieth century, however, inhabitants of the region sometimes had become literally the hunted instead of the hunters.[36]

A violent and prolonged period of colonial conquest and "pacification" caused massive flight from the northern Ovambo flood plain kingdoms of Oukwanyama and the Ombadjas to the middle Ovambo flood plain "wilderness." As the refugees transformed the "wilderness" into landscapes of farms, fields, and villages, colonial officials voiced concerns that the middle flood plain environment was becoming overpopulated and threatened by deforestation and desertification. Unwilling to stop in-migration from Angola because of the increasing demand for migrant labor for Namibian and South African white farms, mines, and industries, the officials cast their eyes on the area east of the Ovambo flood plain and south of the Angolan border: a land they deemed devoid of any settlement and so wild and inhospitable that it was said to be lacking even flies. The presence of the San was taken only to confirm that the area was consummate "wilderness," pristine, untamed, and therefore potentially suitable to settle new refugees from Angola as well as migrants from the "overpopulated" Ovambo flood plain.[37]

The "wildness" of the San in the eyes of colonial officials was underlined by acts of San violence in the 1920s. Some of this may have been a reflection of increased competition between different groups of San and between San groups and Ovambo hunters, herdsmen, or migrants who moved into the wilderness east of the flood plain. In 1927, San reportedly attacked a group of thirty returning Angolan migrant laborers near the border.[38] In

1928, an expedition sent by the colonial administration to survey the east and to dig water holes was forced to turn back because, as its leader explained, "his natives were afraid of the Bushmen."[39] In 1929, a group of San was reported to have robbed two groups of migrant laborers from Angola, killing several. When King Martin of Ondonga sent an armed detail to investigate the incidents, his men clashed with the San culprits in their far eastern hideout, killing their leader. King Martin's men also reported "that the Bushmen had a fight amongst themselves over certain rights and that one man had been killed as a result of a wound from a poisoned arrow and one young girl wounded."[40] In 1930, San from Ongandjera in western Ovamboland northwest of Etosha Pan attacked Uukwaluthi migrant laborers.[41] A 1928 report that highlighted the barrenness of the wilderness east of the Ovambo flood plain suggested that the Bushmen/San must have fled there: "he [the Bushman] has certainly not voluntarily chosen the Sandveld for his home."[42]

The perception of the region's San as living in a state of dislocation is also punctuated by evidence of a crisis in terms of livelihoods. The late 1920s and early 1930s were drought years that triggered famine in the Ovambo flood plain. Colonial officials reported "very rare" occurrences of San men looking for work. In August 1927, for example, seven San men from Angola applied for work as migrant laborers at the recruitment center at Ondangwa. In September 1927, another four "Ondonga-Bushmen" followed suit. Two of the seven San recruits from Angola were diagnosed as having light cases of scurvy, suggesting nutritional stress.[43] It is unclear whether the colonial officials were surprised because they had never heard of San men engaging in migrant labor, or because the San, whom they perceived to lead a simple but idyllic existence, were forced to engage with "civilization"[44]

How could the San, who were an integral part of the "wilderness," possibly be so dramatically affected by a subsistence crisis, forcing them to become robbers and wage laborers? Colonial reports from the 1930s and 1940s explicitly distinguished between the "wild" Bushmen who were nomadic hunter-gatherers and the "tame" Bushmen who were being absorbed in Ovambo culture. Most of the thirteen to sixteen hundred "wild" San who lived east of the Ovambo flood plain were considered to be as "wild" as the Kalahari San, and were thought to "lead a carefree, though at times in drought seasons, a hard life." The 1928 annual report for Ovamboland mentioned that the eastern Ovamboland Bushmen "when they feel the pinch of hunger, move towards the Ovambo settlements, where they generally manage to barter a little grain or other food stuffs."[45] In contrast, the several hundred San in western Ovamboland who had been moved closer to the flood plain to enhance colonial control engaged in agriculture and raised livestock including goats, sheep, cattle, and donkeys and were no longer considered "wild."[46]

If hard times had indeed fallen upon the San as a result of the decline of regional game populations, violence, social dislocation, and physical displacement, then it is the more surprising that their 1920s and 1930s home environment was deemed a "wilderness" despite being neither pristine nor "natural." The "wilderness" east of the flood plain and south of the Angolan-Namibian border contained no remnants of ancient cities or densely populated centers. Even so, it was to a significant extent a domesticated environment. San communities domesticated it through the construction of water holes that formed the basis for settlements, some of which were permanent. Digging and maintaining water holes were extremely labor-intensive. A water hole had to be cleaned of excess sand and litter every year. The Assistant Native Commissioner of Ovamboland, Bourquin, distinguished between San *camps* which were temporary, and San *villages:* in late May 1940, his party failed to locate two temporary San camps and was forced to camp at Omboto where he discovered a "large permanent Bushmen settlement," "the Bushmen village of old Ule, the leader of the group of that area."[47] In a subsequent report, however, although Ule is referred to as a "clan" leader whose authority extended over several San groups in the Omaheke, i.e. they were organized in a chiefdom, its inhabitants were thought to have been "untouched by civilisation and must be considered as typical wild bushmen living in their natural environment."[48] The San waterholes provided stepping stones for Ovambo flood plain migrants' expansion into eastern Ovamboland "wilderness."[49] For example, in 1941 the Assistant Native Commissioner reported:

> When we reached Ombongolo on 29/8/41 we found that the Ukuanyamas had cleaned and enlarged the Bushman waterhole at the spot. . . . at Okulukila a dry Bushman waterhole was found but unfortunately time did not allow us to have it cleaned. . . . At Shikome . . . two small Bushman waterholes about six feet deep were found in use. These were cleaned and enlarged and gave a good supply of water. . . . Further shallow Bushman waterholes were found at Omboto and Oshiti and there is no doubt that it will be possible to sink many waterholes in this locality.[50]

In the same year another report mentioned Kules or Kures [Kudis?] 40–50 miles NWN of Tsintsabis Police Station where there were more or less permanent waterholes, "and where there are always Bushmen. The present leader is Nainabab." Yet another report talked about a San "Chief" in the Omaheke called Hamketeb.[51]

San communities in eastern Ovamboland temporarily abandoned their settlements for the duration of the dry season to follow migrating wildlife. In 1942, the Assistant Native Commissioner reported: "[T]he Omaheke bush is bushmen country. For generations Bushmen have lived here and have established more or less permanent settlements. Each group has its well defined territory ant [*sic*] it moves from waterhole to waterhole within its boundary."[52] Despite the observation that San settlements were permanent and in spite of the explicit association of certain water holes with specific San communities, colonial officials considered "San" water holes to be open access resources. Colonial officials and ethnographers alike maintained that ownership of natural resources was a concept unknown to San culture.[53] In the Ovambo concept of water ownership, a water hole was either owned by the person who dug it, by his or her descendants, or by the person who maintained it. The Ovambo conceptualization meshed with the views of colonial officials, who believed the San were at best "underutilizing" the land, while the Ovambo agro-pastoralists were considered to be able to use the land much more efficiently. In other words, the land use practices employed by the San communities east of the Ovambo flood plain did not qualify as "development." To the contrary, the very presence of "wild" San defined land as "wilderness."

The colonization of the region east of the Ovambo flood plain by Angolan refugees and migrants from the flood plain, legitimized by Ovambo and colonial officials' (re)defining the San as "wild" and their environment as "wilderness," set in motion a process of marginalization of the San as environmental, economic, and social actors. San groups and individuals lost control over much of the eastern "wilderness" and its resources. Matias Kafita, a San, for example, hunted and gathered with his father and other San during his youth but as an adult was merely an assistant to horse-mounted Ovambo hunters.[54]

The structural erosion of San livelihoods by the 1950s became obvious even to colonial officials. Whereas the 1948 annual report for Ovamboland had distinguished "tame" and "wild" Bushmen, the 1951 annual report only used the term "semi-tame" Bushmen in the census, of which it enumerated twenty-five hundred.[55] During the 1952 drought, Ovamboland San were the primary recipients of free food aid, while in 1953, the eastern San temporarily received government assistance, including medical aid at a camp at Omundaunghilo.[56] At the same time, officials recruited the few San remaining in the Namutoni (Etosha) Game Reserve in a project to collect animal bones scattered in the game park. The scheme was initiated in 1950 to allow the San to earn some cash and to supply the bone meal factory at Okahandja. San bone collectors received 2s. 6d. per hundred pounds. By the end of 1950, almost fifty thousand pounds had been purchased.[57] In 1954, however, all San remaining in the park were expelled.[58]

During the 1950s, the San remaining on both sides of the border east of the flood plain received food aid and gifts of tobacco as incentives to assemble at the stations of the Finnish Mission, which in turn resettled them at Okongo and Ekoka in mission villages where they were trained in crop cultivation.[59] A Finnish missionary took Matias Kafita and his family from their Eenhana home first to Okongo and subsequently to Ekoka. When they arrived at Ekoka,

> there was another tribe of San called Ovakwagga !Kung ([they] call themselves Kwagga). My community [was] called Ovagongolo. . . . The Kwagga were like us also in the forest and were hunting animals. The Kwagga left when the [Finnish] Mission came here. At that time [there] were no wild animals around. They gave us the garden; it was for us not for the Mission. We got enough food from the big garden and maize. . . . At the beginning the garden was cultivated as one garden for everybody. When the missionaries found out that we could do the work properly they divided the garden among the people. [There was] only one Kwanyama household headed by Johannes Namidi. He was the village headman of Ekoka. He was looking after the San and was given that task by Eliki [Erik, a Finnish missionary].[60]

It was during this stage in the history of the San in eastern Ovamboland that they became the focus of a surge in academic interest. During 1951, for example, the Portuguese ethnographer Martin Gusinde engaged in research on the region's San and a research group led by Laurence Marshall visited the area. The government's Bushman Commission conducted research in Ovamboland during 1952.[61] By that time, however, the San in the central Angolan-Namibian border region had been reduced to homeless wanderers who owned little more than what they could carry on their backs, and who lived from day to day on what they could hunt, gather, and beg.

That entire ecosystems and individual species, including humans, can historically move back and forth between the categories of domesticated and wild sheds grave doubts on the usefulness of a paradigm that sees environmental change as moving along a gradient (even if only analytically) from a state of pristine wilderness/Nature (or at least from higher degree of "pristineness") to a state of domestication/Culture (or at least a lower level of "pristineness"), with the urban landscape at the lowest point on the continuum. The change is not only construed to be linear, but it is also unilinear and irreversible. This conceptualization in turn results in a paradox whereby environments defined as having been "wilderness" in a more distant or more recent past have in fact been marked and shaped by intensive human use as was the case, for example, at Palenque. And the Palenques are only the tip of the iceberg: the semi-urban and rural humanized environments that sustained similar urban centers must have stretched over much of the modern forest and savanna wilderness landscapes of Central America and Africa, including such an "African Eden" as the Kruger National Park in South Africa.

Notes

1. A good example of the popular image of the simple Bushman "Stone Age" life and its juxtaposition with modern urban life is the film *The Gods Must Be Crazy.* Sahlins stresses that San/Bushmen and other similar communities rejected the "Neolithic revolution," M. Sahlins, *Stone Age Economics* (Chicago: Aldine-Atherton, 1972), p. 27. See also R. Lee, "What Hunters Do for a Living; or How to Make Out on Scarce Resources," in *Man the Hunter,* ed. R. Lee and I. DeVore (Chicago: Aldine, 1968), pp. 30–43.

2. For the "discovery" of stone structures in Central America and Africa, respectively, see, for example, G. S. Stuart and G. E. Stuart, *Lost Kingdoms of the Maya* (Washington, D.C.: National Geographic Society, 1993); and J. H. Venning, "Notes on Southern Rhodesian Ruins in Victoria District," *Journal of the Royal African Society* 7, no. 26 (January 1908): 150–58.

3. For the classic study on the history of the concept of wilderness, see R. Nash, *Wilderness in the American Mind* (1967; New Haven, Conn.: Yale University Press, 1982). Cronon rejects what he calls the human-natural and urban-rural dichotomies, and White points to the "blurring" of the wild-domesticated dichotomy. See W. Cronon, *Nature's Metropolis: Chicago and the Great West* (New York: Norton, 1991), pp. 17–19; and R. White, *The Organic Machine: The Remaking of the Columbia River* (1995; New York: Hill and Wang, 2000), pp. 105–9.

4. On Great Zimbabwe, see M. Hall, *The Changing Past: Farmers, Kings, and Traders in Southern Africa, 200–1860* (Cape Town: D. Philip, 1987), pp. 91–116; and D. N. Beach, *The Shona and Zimbabwe, 900–1850* (1980; Gweru: Mambo Press, 1990), pp. 1–52. On Palenque, Stuart and Stuart, *Lost Kingdoms of the Maya,* pp. 19, 31; and V. Perera and R. D. Bruce, *The Last Lords of Palenque: The Lacandon Indians of the Mexican Rainforest* (1982; Berkeley: University of California Press, 1985), pp. 10–26. On Angkor Wat, see J. Audric, *Angkor and the Khmer Empire* (London: R. Hale, 1972); and D. P. Chandler, *A History of Cambodia* (Boulder, Colo.: Westview Press, 1992).

5. For critiques of the concept of a premodern human-nature "balance," in North America, see, for example, A. Isenberg, *The Destruction of the Bison* (New York: Cambridge University Press, 2000), esp. pp. 2–10. For a similar critique regarding Central America, see for example, J. D. Wingard, "Interactions between Demographic Processes and Soil Resources," in *The Managed Mosaic: Ancient Maya Agriculture and Resource Use,* ed. S. L. Fedick (Salt Lake City: University of Utah Press, 1996), pp. 207–235; and M. J. MacLeod, "Exploitation of Natural Resources in Colonial Central America: Indian and Spanish Approaches," in *Changing Tropical Forests: Historical Perspectives on Today's Challenges in Central and South America,* ed. H. K. Steen and R. P. Tucker (n.p.: Forest History Society, 1992), pp. 31–39. Balée in the latter volume offers a countercritique and argues that Indians did not cause any dramatic biodiversity losses, W. Balée, "Indigenous History and Amazonian Biodiversity," pp. 185–97.

6. Stuart and Stuart, *Lost Kingdoms of the Maya,* pp. 63–64; and D. T. Vlcek, S. Garza de Gonzalez, and E. B. Kurjack, "Contemporary Farming and Ancient Maya Settlements: Some Disconcerting Evidence," in *Pre-Hispanic Maya Agriculture,* ed. P. D. Harrison and B. L. Turner II (Albuquerque: University of New Mexico Press, 1978), pp. 211–223, esp. pp. 218–220.

7. Hartland was one of the first to claim that the temples were the centers of cities and towns; W. A. Hartland, "Maya Settlement Patterns: A Critical Review," in *Archaeological Studies in Middle America,* ed. E. Wyllys Andrews IV et al. (New Orleans: Middle American Research Institute, 1970), p. 37. See also N. P. Dunning, "A Reexamination of Regional Variability in the Pre-Hispanic Agricultural Landscape," in Fedick, *The Managed Mosaic,* pp. 53–91. On the archaeological bias, see E. Graham and D. M. Prendergast, "Maya Urbanism and Ecological Change," in Steen and Tucker, *Changing Tropical Forests,* pp. 102–9; and Stuart and Stuart, *Lost Kingdoms of the Maya,* p. 32.

8. V. Scarborough, "Reservoirs and Watersheds in the Central Maya Lowlands," in Fedick, *The Managed Mosaic,* pp. 304–14. This idea is also very valuable in looking at African precolonial urbanization: Great Zimbabwe, for example, was also not located near a major river.

9. Cronon, *Nature's Metropolis,* pp. 17–19.

10. Graham and Prendergast argue that the concept of "pre-industrial tropical urbanism" sheds new light at the ways environmental change is studied; see Graham and Prendergast, "Maya Urbanism and Ecological Change," pp. 102–9. This hints at the issues at the heart of Cronon's argument, since the nature of precolonial "urbanism" in Central America and Africa in many ways challenges the Eurocentric models of "urbanism": for example, African and Central American urbanism may have been less nucleated.

11. On Tenochtitlán's population and the number of Meso-American ruins, see L. V. Foster, *A Brief History of Central America* (New York: Facts on File, 2000), pp. 20–21. On Chunchumil, see Vlcek, Garza de Gonzalez, and Kurjack, "Contemporary Farming and Ancient Maya Settlement," pp. 212–17. On Nohmul, see K. A. Pyburn, "The Political Economy of Ancient Maya Land Use: The Road to Ruin," in Fedick, *The Managed Mosaic,* pp. 242–43. On Tikal, see Stuart and Stuart, *Lost Kingdoms of the Maya,* p. 32. On Great Zimbabwe, see Hall, *The Changing Past,* pp. 91–116.

12. Angkor Wat: C. Higham, *The Archaeology of Mainland Southeast Asia from 10,000 B.C. to the Fall of Angkor Wat* (Cambridge: Cambridge University Press, 1989), pp. 333, 339–40.

13. D. W. Gade, *Nature and Culture in the Andes* (Madison: University of Wisconsin Press, 1999), p. 52.

14. For in-town garden plots, see Vlcek, Garza de Gonzalez, and Kurjack, "Contemporary Farming and Ancient Maya Settlement," pp. 212–17; and D. E. Puleston, "Terracing, Raised Fields, and Tree Cropping in the Maya Lowlands: A New Perspective on the Geography of Power," in Harris and Turner, *Pre-Hispanic Maya Agriculture,* pp. 226–27, 229–30. See also Dunning, "A Reexamination of Regional Variability in the Pre-Hispanic Agricultural Landscape," pp. 53–91. Dunning defines the ancient communities in the Puuc hill country of Yucatàn and Campeche as "garden cities."

15. Graham and Prendergast, "Maya Urbanism and Ecological Change," pp. 102–9; and R. Hoffmann, "La importancia ecológica y económica de las tecnologías tradicionales en la agri- y silvicultura en áreas de bosque tropical húmido en México," in Steen and Tucker, *Changing Tropical Forests,* 110–22; R. T. Matheny, "Northern Maya Lowland Water Control Systems," in Harrison and Turner, *Pre-Hispanic*

Maya Agriculture, pp. 195, 205; and Puleston, "Terracing, Raised Fields, and Tree Cropping," pp. 225–45. For water harvesting, see also A. Ford, "Critical Resource Use and the Rise of the Classic Period Maya," in Fedick, *The Managed Mosaic,* pp. 297–303, and Scarborough, "Reservoirs and Watersheds in the Central Maya Lowlands," pp. 304–14. For raised fields and irrigation works in the pre-Columbian Andes highlands and lowlands, see J. W. Verano, "Prehistoric Disease and Demography in the Andes," in *Disease and Demography in the Americas,* ed. J. W. Verano and D. H. Ubelaker (Washington, D.C.: Smithsonian Institution Press, 1992), p. 16. For "the myth of the *milpa,*" see S. L. Fedick, "Introduction: New Perspectives on Ancient Maya Agriculture and Resource Use," in Fedick, *The Managed Mosaic,* p. 2. For the degree of environmental management involved in the case of Angkor Wat, see L. Frédéric, *La vie quotidienne dans la Péninsule indochinoise à l'Epoque d'Angkor, 800–1300* (Paris: Hachette Littérature Générale, 1981), pp. 137–38; Higham, *The Archaeology of Mainland Southeast Asia,* pp. 321, 325, 329, 337, 341, 348–52; and Audric, *Angkor and the Khmer Empire,* pp. 125–32.

16. Fedick, "Introduction: New Perspectives on Ancient Maya Agriculture and Resource Use," p. 2; Dunning, "A Reexamination of Regional Variability in the Pre-Hispanic Agricultural Landscape," pp. 53–91; and Ford, "Critical Resource Use," pp. 297–99.

17. Vlcek, Garza de Gonzalez, and Kurjack, "Contemporary Farming," p. 220.

18. P. S. Dunham, "Resource Exploitation and Exchange among the Classic Maya," in Fedick, *The Managed Mosaic,* pp. 320–25.

19. On trade, see Vlcek, Garza de Gonzalez, and Kurjack, "Contemporary Farming," pp. 222–23; and Puleston, "Terracing, Raised Fields, and Tree Cropping," p. 244; Dunham, "Resource Exploitation and Exchange among the Classic Maya," pp. 315–32; Foster, *A Brief History of Central America,* pp. 17, 28, 36–37. On Great Zimbabwe, see Hall, *The Changing Past,* pp. 91–116.

20. B. W. Leyden, M. Brenner, T. Whitmore, J. H. Curtis, D. R. Piperno, and B. H. Dahlin, "A Record of Long- and Short-Term Variation from Northwest Yucatán: Cenote San José Culchacá," in Fedick, *The Managed Mosaic,* pp. 30–49. Fedick stresses that ancient Maya agriculture supported millions of people over centuries in a marginal environment: Fedick, "Introduction: New Perspectives on Ancient Maya Agriculture and Resource Use," p. 10. See also Wingard, "Interactions between Demographic Processes and Soil Resources in the Copán Valley, Honduras," pp. 207–35.

21. S. M. Pierce, "Environmental History of La Selva Biological Station: How Colonization and Deforestation of Sarapiquí Canton, Costa Rica, have Altered the Ecological Context of the Station," in Steen and Tucker, *Changing Tropical Forests,* pp. 40–57, esp. pp. 47–48. See also Konrad in the same volume who argues that the dense forests of the Mayan peninsula formally came to be seen as "uninhabited" only since the late 1800s; H. W. Konrad, "Tropical Forest Policy and Practice during the Mexican Porfiriato, 1876–1910," in Steen and Tucker, *Changing Tropical Forests,* p. 124.

22. S. Rietbergen, ed., *The Earthscan Reader on Tropical Forestry* (London: Earthscan, 1993), pp. 1–2; and S. G. Boyce, *Landscape Forestry* (New York: Wiley, 1995), p. vii.

23. J. S. Adams and T. O. McShane, *The Myth of Wild Africa: Conservation without Illusion* (1992; Berkeley: University of California Press, 1996), pp. 1–13. Sheperd,

Shanks, and Hobley point out that Africa has two-thirds of the world's open tropical forests and two-thirds of its shrub land. They also add that in Africa it is often impossible to distinguish between woodland and farmland because, for example, land moves between the two categories (for example fallow lands) and because a herdsman effectively considers woodland to be his farm. G. Sheperd, E. Shanks, and M. Hobley, "Management of Tropical and Subtropical Dry Forests," in Rietbergen, *The Earthscan Reader on Tropical Forestry,* pp. 107–36, esp. pp. 107 and 112. R. P. Neumann, *Imposing Wilderness: Struggles over Livelihood and Nature Preservation in Africa* (Berkeley: University of California Press, 1998). On the Kruger Park, see J. Carruthers, *The Kruger Park: A Social and Political History* (Pietermaritzburg: University of Natal Press, 1995). On the Makuleke and the forced removals, see B. de Villiers, *Land Claims and National Parks: The Makuleke Experience* (Pretoria: Human Sciences Research Council, 1999), pp. 45–57.

24. See interviews with the author: Julius Abraham, Olupito, 15 and 16 June 1993; Petrus Shanika, Oshiteyatemo, 17 June 1993; and Mathias Malaula, Onandjaba, 15 June 1993; E. Kreike, *Re-Creating Eden: Land Use, Environment, and Society in Southern Angola and Northern Namibia* (Westport, Conn.: Heinemann, 2004), chaps. 2, 4, and 7.

25. See interviews with the author: Julius Abraham, Olupito, 15 and 16 June 1993; Petrus Shanika, Oshiteyatemo, 17 June 1993; and Mathias Malaula, Onandjaba, 15 June 1993; and Kreike, *Re-Creating Eden,* chaps. 2, 4, and 7.

26. See especially D. M. Lima, *A campanha dos cuamatos: Contado por um sodado expedicionàrio* (Lisbon: Livraria Ferreira, 1908). See also A. Wülfhorst, *Von Hexen und Zaubern: Bilder aus dem Leben der heidnischen Amboleute in Süd-West-Afrika* (Wuppertal and Barmen: n.p., 1935), pp. 6, 13, and 17; Archives Générales de la Congrégation du Saint-Esprit, Paris (henceforth AGCSSp), Duparquet 1879 journal, entries 12–14, 19–20 August and 5 September 1879; P. J. Veth, *Daniel Veth's Reizen in Angola* (Haarlem: H. D. Tjeenk Willink, 1887), pp. 340–41; P. Möller, *Journey in Africa through Angola, Ovamboland and Damaraland* (Cape Town: C. Struik, 1972), pp. 110–12.

27. See E. Kreike, "Hidden Fruit: A Social Ecology of Fruit Trees in Namibia and Angola, 1880s–1990s," in *Social History and African Environments,* ed. W. Beinart and J. McGregor (Oxford: James Currey, 2003), pp. 27–42. For Latin America, see especially Graham and Prendergast, "Maya Urbanism and Ecological Change," pp. 102–9; and Pierce, "Environmental History of La Selva Biological Station," p. 53; Puleston, "Terracing, Raised Fields, and Tree Cropping," pp. 226–30. See also Gade, *Nature and Culture in the Andes,* pp. 61, 63.

28. AGCSSp, Duparquet 1879 journal, 8 August, 9, 20 September 1879; Duparquet 1882 journal, 14 July 1882; J. de Oliveira Ferreira Diniz, *Negocios indigenas: Relatório do ano de 1913* (Luanda: Imprensa Nacional, [1913]), pp. 14–15. For a more detailed discussion, see Kreike, *Re-Creating Eden,* chap. 3.

29. W. G. Clarence-Smith, *Slaves, Peasants, and Capitalists in Southern Angola, 1840–1926* (Cambridge: Cambridge University Press, 1979), p. 75; interviews: Paulus Haifeke, Oshomokwiyu, 28 April 1993, Paulus Nandenga, Oshomokwiyu, 28 April 1993, Kulaumoni Haifeke, Oshomokwiyu, 11 May 1993, and Julius Abraham, Olupito, 15–16 June 1993; AGCSSp, Duparquet, 1879 journal, 20, 22 August, 8, 11, 21 September 1879.

30. Luiz de Mello e Athayde, "O perigo de despovoamento de Angola," pp. 229–30, Arquivo Historico Ultramarino, Lisbon, Sala 8, Praca 115, Angola, Prejuizos causados pela guerra de 1914–18, Luanda, 14 August 1919. For more details, see Kreike, *Re-Creating Eden,* chaps. 3–4. Kjekhus describes similar processes in late nineteenth-century Tanzania: H. Kjekhus, *Ecology Control and Economic Development in East African History: The Case of Tanganyika, 1850–1950* (London: Heinemann, 1970), pp. 6–7, 126–80.

31. See, for example, J. Vansina, *Paths in the Rainforest: Toward a History of Political Tradition in Equatorial Africa* (Madison: University of Wisconsin Press, 1990), p. 46.

32. E. Wilmsen, *Land Filled with Flies: A Political Economy of the Kalahari* (Chicago: University of Chicago Press, 1989); R. J. Gordon, *The Bushmen Myth: The Making of a Namibian Underclass* (Boulder, Colo.: Westview Press, 1993), pp. 15–43. For a classic study of the San, see R. B. Lee, *The !Kung San: Men, Women, and Work in a Foraging Society* (Cambridge: Cambridge University Press, 1979).

33. Kreike, *Re-Creating Eden,* chap. 2.

34. In 1928, King Martin of Ondonga in the southeastern flood plain employed Bushmen as hunters, messengers, and spies, National Archives of Namibia, Native Affairs Ovamboland (hereafter NAN, NAO), 18 f. 11/1 (I), Annual Report Ovamboland 1928.

35. Cf. Isenberg, *The Destruction of the Bison,* who argues that the Plains Indians contributed to the demise of the bison; and Foster, *A Brief History of Central America,* p. 10, who links the extinction of large mammals in Central America to Indian overhunting.

36. Kreike, *Re-Creating Eden,* chaps. 2–3, 7.

37. Ibid., chap. 7.

38. NAN, NAO 36 f. 26/8 (i), District Surgeon Ondangwa, Monthly Reports August–September 1927.

39. NAN, NAO 17 f. 10/3 (i), Eedes to Hahn, Namakunde, 9 April 1928.

40. NAN, NAO 11 f. 5/9, Officer Commanding Native Affairs Ovamboland to Clarke, Ondangwa, 6 June 1929. See also NAO 18 f. 11/1 (i), Annual Report Ovamboland 1928.

41. NAN, NAO 18 f. 11/1 (iii), Monthly Reports Ovamboland, May–June 1930.

42. NAN, Angola Boundary Commission and Kunene Water Commissions, vol. 1 (iii), W. Volkmann, 30 October 1928, "Report on the Agricultural and Political Conditions at The Angola Boundary."

43. NAN, NAO 36 f. 26/8 (i), District Surgeon Ondangwa, Monthly Reports August–September 1927.

44. Lee argues that the San and hunter-gatherers in general are much less vulnerable to subsistence crises because their main food consists of wild vegetables and fruits which he considers a "stable" resource; Lee, "What Hunters Do for a Living," pp. 30–43.

45. NAN, NAO 18 f. 11/1 (i), Annual Report Ovamboland 1928. The 1934 annual report also emphasizes that Bushmen acquired grain, beans, and tobacco, NAO 19, f. 11/1 (vii). A 1948 report stated that the San suffered from venereal disease, and "habitual coughs" with a high death rate, but added that "[they] seem happy and care free," NAO 61, f. 12/2 (I), Annual Report Ovamboland 1948.

46. NAN, NAO 20 f. 11/1 (xi), Annual Report Ovamboland 1938. For "wild" and "tame" Bushmen, see also NAO 20 f. 11/1 (xv), Annual Report Ovamboland 1942, and NAO 61 f. 12/2 (I), Annual Report Ovamboland 1948.

47. NAN, NAO 10 f. 5/7/1, Assistant Native Commissioner (ANC) to Native Commissioner Ovamboland (NCO), Oshikango, 30 July 1940, "Report on Development Work undertaken in Eastern Ukuanyama during 1940," and NAO 20 f. 11/1 (xiii), Monthly Report Ovamboland, May 1940.

48. NAN, NAO 20 f. 11/1 (xv), Annual Report Ovamboland 1942.

49. A 1928 sketch map indicates eight locations with water holes between Ohinengena (just east of the inhabited zone of Oukwanyama at the time) and Otufima, including one location in Angola. A San settlement is explicitly indicated at Nehova Pan. Some of these water holes may have been dug by San and/or by herdsmen. See map accompanying NAN, NAO 17 f. 10/3 (i), Acting Union Government Representative to Officer Commanding Native Affairs Ovamboland, Namakunde, 25 February 1928. On a sketch map dating from 1932, a San water hole and settlement are indicated at Ombongola, south of beacon 40. Another San water hole is indicated between beacons 37 and 38. A third water hole is indicated near Outafima between beacons 29 and 30, i.e. on the easternmost route of the Oshimolo Trail. See NAO 17 f. 10/3 (i), Officer Commanding Oshikango, Oshikango, [date illegible] March 1932.

50. NAN, NAO 10 f. 5/7/1, ANC to NCO, Oshikango, 6 September 1941, "Proposed Extension of Ukuanyama up to and including Ombongolo Muramba."

51. NAN, NAO 21 f. 12/1/2, NCO to Deputy Commissioner South African Police, Windhoek, 31 December 1941, and Station Commander of the South African Police (SAP) to District Commander SAP Omaruru, Tsintsabis, 20 February 1942.

52. The ANC added that "[n]o reliable information could be obtained from the local Bushmen who do not appear to travel far afield but remain in more or less well defined areas in the Omaheke country." NAN, NAO 10 f. 5/7/1, ANC to NCO, Oshikango, 10 July 1942, "Proposed Extension of Ukuanyama Area: General Report Development Work Eastern Ukuanayama."

53. NAN, NAO 10 f. 5/7/1, ANC to NCO, Oshikango, 8 October 1942. Lee acknowledges that the Dobe-San of the Botswana Kalahari Desert were not truly nomadic and notes that main San camps were located at permanent water holes: Lee, "What Hunters Do for a Living," pp. 31, 35.

54. Matias Kafita, interview by the author, Ekoka laKula, 23 February 1993. See also Moses Kakoto, interview by the author, Okongo, 17 February 1993.

55. NAN, NAO 61 f. 12/2 (I), Annual Reports Ovamboland 1948 and 1951.

56. NAN, NAO 60 f. 12/1–2 (i), Quarterly Report Ovamboland, 4th Quarter 1952, and NAO 64 f. 19/1 (ii), Medical Officer Ovamboland, Monthly Reports August–September 1953.

57. NAN, NAO 59 f. 9/15, NCO to Sec. SWA, Ondangwa, 8 December 1950, and NCO to Station Commander SAP Namutoni, Ondangwa, 14 January 1950; Station Commander SAP Namutoni to NCO, Namutoni, 20 December 1950, and Director Agriculture to Sec. SWA, Windhoek, 22 October 1952.

58. NAN, NAO 61 f. 19/2 (ii), Annual Report Ovamboland 1953.

59. Interviews: Matias Kafita, Ekoka laKula, 23 February 1993, and Moses Kakoto, Okongo, 17 February 1993.

60. Matias Kafita, interview, Ekoka laKula, 23 February 1993.

61. NAN, NAO 60 f. 12/1 (ii), Quarterly Reports Oukwanyama, April–June and July–September 1951. On the Bushman Commission, NAO 106 Diary NCO 1949–1952, entries 30 July, 2 and 3 August 1952.

9

"Paris et le désert français"

Urban and Rural Environments in Post–World War II France

Sara B. Pritchard

Paris was no longer just the greatest city in France.
By 1789, *it was already France itself.*

—Alexis de Tocqueville, *L'Ancien Régime et la Révolution.* Quoted by Jean-François Gravier in the opening epigraph to *Paris et le désert français* (1947)

Recent events have shown how concentration, which taints the economic, social, and political life of our country, is a danger for all of France. . . . It is fundamental and urgent to rebalance (rééquilibrer) *France. Yet we must avoid the same vice for which we reproach the national capital: that is, creating polarized regions around a regional capital, which end up playing the role of a harmful devitalizing force outside its zone of influence.*

The geographic situation of Provence and the development of the great Rhône corridor require an intimate cooperation among all regions that are interested in the development of a major north-south axis for the Common Market as well as its extensions into Africa.

—Antoine Pinay, "Une alliance d'avenir à l'échelle de l'Europe: Le Grand Delta" (1968).

In 1947, Jean-François Gravier, a recently minted geography Ph.D., published Paris et le désert françaisa slim volume on the political and economic status of contemporary France. In it, Gravier condemned the gross inequalities between Paris and the rest of the country, what he called "the French desert." While Paris was urban, powerful, rich, and "modern," much of the rest of France was rural, stagnant, poor, and "backward." Consequently, the provinces sapped the country's wealth and vitality. Gravier's book was both widely read by the general public and influential within government circles. Indeed, his memorable characterization of the French periphery as a "desert" has become incorporated into political and popular discourse as shorthand for the related problems of regional economic disparities and the excessive power of Paris.

Gravier's analysis was rooted in long-standing critiques of centralization and cities, but it reflected the particular state of post–World War II France. Gravier, a geographer, employed a spatial lens in his analysis of the country's contemporary political economy. By doing so, he exposed the complicated spatial politics of post-1945 France. Immediate postwar reconstruction might have restored electricity to homes and repaired the country's war-torn industries, but these measures had not necessarily resolved the economic inequalities between the center and the periphery. Yet the Cold War, decolonization, and European integration made these issues urgent. Could France regain its status as a world leader if most of the country was weak and drained its overall potential?

In response to these concerns, the French state began to implement reforms to promote regionalization over the next few decades. Between 1945 and 1964, political and economic reforms began to modify the country's geographical "disequilibrium." In the process, the centralized model of the French state became increasingly contested, eventually resulting in the creation of twenty-two official "regions," or interdepartmental polities. On the economic front, the broader project of *l'aménagement du territoire* (literally, territorial development, but usually translated as regional planning) soon replaced the more narrow demands of postwar reconstruction. *L'aménagement du territoire* was part of a national mission and therefore aimed to meet regional needs within France, but it did so within the context of the emerging European Economic Community (EEC).

Regionalization both as political reform and as restructuring of economic relations reshaped France's Rhône River. In fact, the regionalization of the Rhône promised to help solve the problem of the French "desert" in at least three ways. First, the Rhône became a locus of regionalism and regional identity. By the late 1960s, a regionalist vision of the Rhône coexisted with a national and nationalist perspective that had been forged in the wake of World War II.[1] Second, the emergence of *l'aménagement du territoire* within France reframed the river's role within the national economy. Regional economic development, which was rooted in postwar reconstruction and began to take off in the mid-1950s, aimed to correct the "backward" state of the provinces. The Rhône served as a potent potential vehicle of regional regeneration. Its waters could be tapped, harnessed, and turned into economic rewards. Indeed, the lower Rhône valley was one of the first places where a national policy of regional economic development was tested. Finally, the Rhône's emergent "regional" character was not limited to its relationship to the rest of France. It was also connected to the whole of Europe. After the creation of the Common Market in 1957, developing the Rhône aimed to strengthen the role of southeastern France within Europe. Decolonization intensified the importance of this transnational, pan-European context. This was particularly true in the southeastern part of the country as the loss of empire weakened regional metropoles such as Marseille, which had been dependent on the greater Mediterranean. As the anchor of *le Grand Delta,* a developed Rhône promised to restore the greater Rhône region and France itself.

In the process, these efforts attempted to cultivate a new relationship between cities and countryside. Despite attempts to solve the related problems of political centralization and economic disequilibrium, they persisted, albeit in new forms. Regional metropoles threatened to reproduce Paris on a small scale. The French thought that they could design away the central position of the city, granting more power to the countryside. Yet in the end, their success came from redistributing power to regional cities. Cities and countryside needed one another and despite creative attempts to disentangle them, the French were not able to escape that central fact. Furthermore, regional cities and their hinterlands might yield other benefits. Healthy regions within France might ensure the country's place within a newly integrated Europe.

The urban and the rural thus played important roles in the Rhône's respatialization from an undifferentiated territory within a nation to a constituent region of a nation. Both politically and economically, regionalization embodied a critique of Paris. As France's quintessential city, Paris embodied centralized political control and excessive economic power. Paris epitomized the dislocation of power from place. Rooted in longer critiques of centralization and the perceived threat of cities, postwar critics like Gravier attempted to correct this unequal geography of power through state planning and development. In the process, ideas of the nation and the region were partly articulated through the urban and the rural. Moreover, contemporaries believed that the future of France depended on ensuring the proper distribution of and relations between urban and rural places.

After receiving his doctorate, Jean-François Gravier initially served as a bureaucrat in the wartime Vichy government. He joined the General Secretary of Youth in 1941 and the Alexis Carrel Foundation two years later. After the war, he joined the Ministry of Reconstruction at the age of thirty where he remained from 1945 to 1949. In 1950, three years after the publication of *Paris et le désert français,* he became a member of the state's economic and technological planning commission, the *Commissariat général au Plan,* where he worked for fifteen years. The *Plan* gave Gravier an opportunity to put his ideas into practice. He hoped to use its activities in order to promote the health of regions as counterweights to Paris. During his tenure there, Gravier was also member of the Governing Council for Regional Economic Development from 1959 to 1964.

As Gravier's own career illustrates, French geographers became more involved in the formulation of political-economic policy within the government after World War II. Gravier advocated an active government role in shaping development. Through planning and policies, the state might revive regions suffering from stagnation. Criticizing capitalism, Gravier argued that a liberal economy and laissez-faire policy had contributed to regional disparities. State oversight might therefore correct such inequalities. In particular, concentration in a few urban areas exacerbated this monopolization. Big cities dominated small ones and eventually incorporated them. After the war, a rural exodus helped to maintain the preeminence of Paris as rural populations declined and urbanization accelerated. In response to these problems, Gravier proposed state-sponsored regional development to revive the provinces, diminish the power of Paris, and ensure the balanced development of France.[2] His postwar critique of the existing geography of power, and the relationship he drew between the nation, region, urban, and rural, built upon existing discourses criticizing both centralization and cities dating back to the late eighteenth and nineteenth centuries.

In *L'Ancien Régime et la Révolution,* Alexis de Tocqueville argued that by the early days of the French revolution, Paris "was already France itself."[3] His equivalence of Paris and the nation alluded to the centralization of the French state. Yet a centralized state was a historical product and a relatively recent one at that. Regional centers such as Montpellier and Lyon, which had arguably rivaled Paris during the early modern era, became increasingly subject to the oversight of the nascent absolute monarchy. While the French Revolution enacted significant changes in political order, the revolutionary legacy shared with its monarchical predecessor a propensity for centralization. During the first month of the Revolution, for instance, all municipalities across France were placed under one common law. As one leading scholar has put it, the largely verbal absolutism of the French kings was somewhat ironically achieved through the Revolution of 1789. Yet not all revolutionaries agreed with this change. Girondins, whose political support came from the countryside, supported greater local liberty. In the end, however, it was the Jacobins, advocates of centralization and statism, who succeeded in implementing their political vision in postrevolutionary France.[4]

In addition to consolidating political centralization, the French Revolution also fixed the terms of the debate over centralization and decentralization. It pitted unity and equality against decentralized power and autonomy. In other words, "by assuming an opposition between unity and equality on the one hand and local liberty on the other, the Revolution ensured that local democracy lagged far behind national democracy." According to this view, the creation of alternative political territorialities such as regions with substantial rights and responsibilities of their own threatened a return to the provincial federalism of the *ancien régime,* which the revolution had just overturned. This argumentative framework has had an enduring legacy. Between 1789 and the Third Republic (1870–1940), legislators rarely challenged the Jacobin principles of centralization, "which put the concerns of national unity and the demands of equality before the law first and the Girondin desire for local liberty second."[5] One of the legacies of 1789 was, then, resistance to decentralization.

These alternative political visions did not entirely disappear in either the nineteenth or the twentieth century. Clemenceau proposed establishing regions in the early 1920s. Yet it was only after World War II that a more sustained critique of centralization emerged when the dramatic post-1945 economic growth known as *les trentes glorieuses* ("The Thirty Glorious Years") exacerbated France's "disequilibrium." A number of agricultural and industrial problems particularly plagued the west and south of France. In time, an unequal economy, uneven rates of growth, and the undeniable reality of regional differences eventually helped to undermine this geography of concentrated political and economic power.[6]

As Gravier's book attested, these disparities sparked the interest of geographers, planners, and politicians.[7] Postwar social scientists began to critique traditional political authority and to develop an alternative spatial language of power, which favored the regional and the local. They also began to question the Jacobin rationality that had driven centralization and a unified national administration.[8] Geographers such as Gravier joined a number of state agencies involved in assessing, analyzing, and solving disparities within a supposed national body. Their spatial approach to problems of economy, politics, and society became incorporated into state programs.

Yet national politicians expressed fears about undermining France as a nation if they enacted substantial political reform and supported the creation of regions as intermediaries between the communes and departments, and the national government. In 1963, Michel Debré, one of de Gaulle's former prime ministers, confessed a "fear of seeing competition from twenty regional parliaments, which might be capable of preparing the disintegration of the nation with the complicity of European organizations."[9] That regions were now framed within a European context only seemed to further threaten national autonomy.

Consequently, reform proceeded slowly and was not without complications. According to critics, the French state, embodied in Paris itself, had excessive power. Local democracy and regionalization were responses to these excesses. They aimed to alter the existing geography of power. But some feared that enacting political reform might undermine national unity and thus threaten "France" itself. As we have seen, this fear had restrained the pace and extent of political reform for several centuries. Moreover, even if regions were created, regional inequalities had the potential to mirror national inequalities. Because regional city centers, *villes-pôles,* played a structuring role for the region in which they were located, they might end up dominating their regions as much as Paris dominated France. Regions could therefore not escape the pull of cities, even if those cities were not Paris.[10]

Despite these concerns, this spatial representation and location of political authority began to shift. In 1964, the national government created twenty-two official "regions," polities that mediated between the communes and departments, and the national government located in Paris. Creating the "region" was essentially a socio-political project: to reorganize power and thereby alter the social order along more horizontal lines. Its early powers were limited, but reforms in 1982, following the Socialist electoral victory the previous year, began to transfer more substantial powers to the local and regional levels. One scholar has argued that these political reforms embodied a shift from "*le* territoire" to "*les* territoires," or a shift from a singular national territory to a less centralized, more fragmented, and less uniform set of territorialities.[11]

Yet this shift had implications outside France. If regions became the building blocks of the European Economic Community, then they could prove as important as, if not more important than the nation-state. *L'aménagement du territoire* therefore attempted to remedy the differences between internal national territorialities that Gravier had identified.[12] Proponents of *l'aménagement du territoire* argued that the stakes of failing to do so were high. Regions needed to become efficient and productive, or else other regions, whether in France or across Europe, might leave them behind.[13] Effective *aménagement du territoire* could improve regions, but it could also secure national interests. Here, regional, national, and international concerns intertwined.

Embedded within Gravier's critique of Paris was another discourse rooted in the nineteenth century: a critique of cities and their detrimental influence on France and its citizenry. According to this perspective, urban life and urban environments posed a number of serious threats to the individual, the human body, and the social body. These concerns reflected the industrialization and urbanization that France underwent between the early nineteenth and mid-twentieth centuries. These anxieties found expression in diverse sources. For instance, many of the novels of Emile Zola's Rougon-Macquart series such as *Germinal* deal with the detrimental effect of city life on people in general and particularly on those moving from the country to the city. Politicians and police, social theorists and socialists, doctors and public health officials, activists and architects dealt with the "problem" of the city in various ways.

A number of issues sparked their concern. The conveniences and pleasures of the city—by the late nineteenth century, these included electricity, cafés, and department stores—concealed its dangers. The seeming rise in criminality over the nineteenth century suggested a moral decline associated with urbanization. Physicians and social scientists had even identified a national disease, *dégénérescence,* a medico-moral condition of physical deterioration paralleled by moral and intellectual decline. Amid these anxieties over the possible devolution of French society, crime and criminality became particular preoccupations. Higher crime rates, new crimes, and new kinds of criminals all seemed to demonstrate the validity of theories about the degenerative powers of the city as well as the pervasiveness of decline. Modernity and urbanity were thus afflicted by pathological behavior, but they had also helped to create it.[14]

Similarly, just as cities bred social pathology and degeneration, critics also argued that they created physical pathology and degeneration. As in many cities in western Europe and the United States, an outbreak of cholera struck Paris and other large cities in France in 1832. Poverty, poor labor conditions, and urbanization had helped to create an ideal disease environment and compounded the impacts of the epidemic. Subsequent outbreaks indicated that urban spaces were model breeding grounds for illness, particularly communicable diseases. Public health reforms attempted to respond to disease and, to varying extents, its economic and social conditions. Furthermore, it was not only the threats to the physical body which diseases posed that worried some contemporaries. The urban mind was also at risk. According to critics, the dark underside of the city produced fatigue, neurasthenia, restlessness, and *ennui* among the upper class while workers and the poor easily fell prey to vice.[15] Contemporary critics thus lamented the social, health, and moral problems created by urban environments.

Public health programs indicated how the state intervened in an attempt to manage a modern, industrial society, but urban reform was another method of social control over the seeming dangers of urban environments. Georges Haussmann, prefect of the Seine department from 1853 to 1869, epitomized the transformation of urban space for socio-political objectives. Just months after the establishment of the conservative Second Empire, which had replaced the short-lived republic founded after the revolution of 1848, Haussmann developed big plans for the transformation of Paris. Backed by Emperor Napoleon III, Haussmann hoped to transform the capital's infrastructure. During his tenure, Haussmann oversaw a wide range of projects to remake the physical environment of the city. His program laid out expansive sewer networks, supplied much of the city with running water, built wide boulevards that radiated out from central Paris, and planted trees. In the process of modernizing the basic infrastructure of urban life, Haussmannization razed some of the city's poorest neighborhoods while filling the pocketbooks of wealthy developers.[16]

Coming on the heels of 1848, replacement of urban slums with new buildings and modern facilities aimed to increase control over the city's population that had participated in France's most recent revolution. Surveillance and discipline were inscribed into new urban spaces such as the grand boulevard of the Champs-Elysées. Previous revolutions had shown how easy it was for rebels to build barricades across narrow streets. Expansive boulevards were much harder to block, thereby facilitating police and military repression of urban riots. In part, the modernization of nineteenth-century Paris thus attempted to squelch revolutionary potential through the remaking of urban space. Municipal infrastructure and urban reform served as technopolitics of state control under the Second Empire.[17]

Fears about criminality, disease, and urban space suggested how contemporaries worried about the detrimental influence of cities on political, cultural, and intellectual conditions. Paired with this discourse of urban degeneration was an idealization of rural life. The Vichy regime epitomized the glorification of agriculture and the peasant during the 1940s, but it was rooted in the longer criticism of urbanity. Vichy favored agricultural development, shifting state policies from industrial to agricultural objectives. These interests framed Vichy's view of the countryside and underlay its policies towards economic development nationally. The *Délégation générale de l'équipement national,* arguably the first government agency for *l'aménagement du territoire,* was created by Vichy in 1943. It criticized the dominating influence of Paris and large industrial cities in the north and northeast, which had swallowed up smaller towns. The agency aimed to achieve a greater harmony of relations between cities and the countryside by promoting certain kinds of economic development. It promoted a reconfigured relationship between the urban and the rural following the industrialization and urbanization of the nineteenth century. Indicative of this view, Vichy also established youth organizations to remove the country's children from the dangers of city life. While urban environments might contaminate, pollute, and degenerate, the countryside promised renewal and regeneration.[18]

Gravier's *Paris et le désert français* was published three years after liberation and the end of the Vichy regime. While many French sought to break ties with Vichy after the war because of the opprobrious legacy of collaboration, historians have emphasized some of the continuities between Vichy and the Fourth Republic. Gravier's critique represented one such continuity. His condemnation of Paris reflected a century-long angst over the detrimental influence of the urban and a celebration of the restorative possibilities of the rural. The overall "health" of France was tied to the proper relationship between Paris and the countryside. After World War II, however, new articulations of these older issues emerged as modernization and industrialization intensified, urbanization and suburbanization increased, and immigration and repatriation altered the country's demography.

After 1945, regional economic development echoed some of these older tensions between cities and their hinterlands. Urbanization became one of the main preoccupations of French regional policy, especially because "urban" France was a relatively recent phenomenon. It was not until 1930 that at least half of France's population lived in cities. This shift to an urban majority occurred a full century after a similar shift in England and fifty years later than in Germany. Concern over urbanization reflected tensions between Paris and the rest of France, but regional centers were both problems and solutions to this concentration. Regional "pole cities" might balance Paris, but they threatened to dominate their surrounding areas. Planning authorities therefore attempted to create a harmonious provincial urban structure and to plan an appropriate urban hierarchy.

In 1950, the government established and funded the *Plan national d'aménagement du territoire.*[19] Its first report defined "large provincial agglomerations, which exercise a true directing role in the economic and social life of a regional or multiregional zone of influence, thus avoiding all generalized recourse to the capital." It identified eight of these *métropoles régionales,* also called *métropoles d'équilibre.* The two most important regional metropoles were Lyon and Marseille, followed by Bordeaux, Lille, Strasbourg, Toulouse, Nantes, and Nancy. Below Paris, these eight cities formed the highest level of the urban hierarchy. Filling in the rest of the hierarchy, the plan listed ten "regional centers" and then specified three subsequent levels of towns. Some neighboring cities might be combined into greater centers: Marseille, Aix-en-Provence, and the Rhône Delta were the heart of the Mediterranean southeast while Lyon and St.-Etienne were the center of the non-Mediterranean southeast.

The creation of *le Grand Delta* in southeastern France embodied the regionalization of the country. As the heart of *le Grand Delta,* the Rhône River played a central role in regional economic renewal. *Le Grand Delta* referred not only to the river's delta itself, but usually also included the entire Rhône valley. Most advocates conceived of the delta even more broadly than this already loose interpretation of river geography. In their view, the delta stretched across the entire French Mediterranean—from Perpignan to Nice—and reached inland as far north as Lyon.

In December 1966, businessmen, politicians, and public leaders founded an association for *le Grand Delta,* officially called the *Association pour le développement économique et social du Sud-Est français.* Its *conseil d'administration* was made up of representatives from departmental *conseils généraux,* regional economic expansion committees, chambers of agriculture, ports, and regional development companies, among others. The association's objective was to coordinate and promote economic activities, planning, and development in the three neighboring regions created by the 1964 law: the Rhône-Alpes, Languedoc-Roussillon, and Provence–Côte d'Azur.[20] This association thus promoted southeastern France to businesses and politicians within France and across Europe. The association was essentially a well-funded marketing campaign, advertising the idea of *le Grand Delta* and its rich potential for economic growth and regional development. A journal, *Delta: Revue d'Action Régionale,* marketed the idea through educational and promotional articles as well as advertisements from towns and departments lobbying for new business.[21] In June 1972, the association sponsored an exposition for over twelve hundred business leaders from across Europe, at which individual communes, departments, and regions promoted themselves by arranging wine tastings, tours, and other activities for attendees.[22]

State elites and business leaders adopted *le Grand Delta* as their conceptual framework for southeastern France in order to plan its future.[23] To find rational solutions to the problems that southeastern France faced, politicians and planners needed to consider the entire area together. Consequently, this interregional cooperation and "solidarity" mediated between the nation and region.[24] Some argued that *le Grand Delta* marked the creation of "an entirely new regional entity, deliberately conceived in a European context and on the scale of an enlarged European Community."[25]

Le Grand Delta thus recast the geography of regional planning within France and across Europe. In France, the twenty-two regions that had recently been created could be recombined into eight interregional groups, or "zones of studies and territorial development." *Le Grand Delta* was one of those eight interregional groups. Similarly, EEC experts envisioned regional *découpage* ("cutting up") of their member countries.[26] Both France and the EEC had adopted, then, a regional approach to development. Yet within France, the regional had become interregional while within the context of Europe, the regional could potentially cross national boundaries. The new *politique* of regionalization could therefore work within or it might undermine national sovereignty.

The periphery of France did not necessarily seem to be, then, "the desert" of Gravier's book. In fact, the *Grand Delta* association and its supporters saw places like the greater Rhône valley as a promising solution to the country's postwar challenges. They highlighted a number of the region's promising resources—from the human and environmental to the technological and geopolitical.

Unlike other provincial areas of France, which suffered from population declines and rural exodus, southeastern France had experienced remarkable demographic growth and vitality during the 1960s. In fact, all three southeastern regions had demographic growth rates between 1962 and 1968 that exceeded that of Paris. During these years, the population of Paris rose 9 percent, but Provence–Côte d'Azur grew by an astonishing 17 percent while the other two regions each increased by an impressive 10 percent. Large provincial cities such as Marseille had even higher rates of growth than these regional averages.

In addition to its competitive growth rates, the total population of southeastern France made it a formidable rival to the capital. While the population of Paris was slightly larger than that of *le Grand Delta* in 1962, the situation had been reversed by 1968. The southeast now had a "critical population mass" that made it competitive Europe-wide.[27] Much of this growth was the result of decolonization. The repatriation of French citizens from former colonies as well as increased immigration contributed to the country's overall population increase. One Lyon politician recommended even more growth, so that the area could compete with other European regions such as northern Germany. Yet such growth had to be carefully managed, he warned, since it might exacerbate regional demographic inequalities.[28]

This warning indicated concern over the relationship between the urban and rural within regional economic development. State reports asserted that the "success of developing the Rhône corridor and the Mediterranean coastline in the future depends in large part on solving the excessive retardation of the infrastructure and equipment of the two metropoles of Lyon and Marseille." To ensure their roles as *métropoles d'équilibre* against the centralizing vortex of Paris, both cities had to be developed, equipped, and made more functional.[29] Regional cities needed more autonomy, resources, and control over the destinies of their surrounding hinterlands in order to balance Paris.

These demographic resources aided the southeast's competitiveness, but water, and specifically the Rhône's water, was the region's greatest asset. Creating *le Grand Delta* could reverse the southeast's marginality. "Nature has given us a magnificent instrument," one author avowed. "It is the Rhône, and it has to be said that until the present, it has not played the role that it could have."[30] Furthermore, the Rhône's potential seemed infinite. The state described the "almost limitless quantities" of water resources along the river. Moreover, regional development companies had diverted some of the Rhône's waters, thus extending the river's benefits beyond the narrow confines of the river valley to the entire French Mediterranean littoral.[31] The river's potential value for transportation and communication, economic sectors critical to the regeneration of southeastern France, was tremendous.[32] Deep-water ports, hydraulic engineering projects on key rivers, and large waterways had created a "fluvial axis" into the heart of Europe. Advocates of development even compared southeastern France to California, except that unlike parched California, the Rhône ensured that "la Californie européenne" had abundant water.[33]

In highlighting the potential rewards of the area's demographic and natural resources, advocates of *le Grand Delta* did not hope for blind, directionless economic expansion. They had three specific goals for what regional economic development was supposed to do. First, it should revive Marseille and the city's surrounding area, a part of the country that had been hit hard by decolonization. Marseille was France's primary Mediterranean port and one with a very long history. For centuries, it had connected France not only to the rest of Europe, but also to global trade networks. Lyon and Marseille had once rivaled, if not surpassed Paris in importance. Power had shifted to the north and specifically to Paris. Marseille's former role served as a reminder, however, that the centralizing role of Paris was historical, not inevitable.

Of all parts of France, the loss of the country's North African colonies hit Marseille particularly hard. As one author put it, "Given that Marseille no longer has an empire in front of it, that it no longer has North Africa, that it no longer has French territories on the other side of the Mediterranean Sea, it is therefore necessary that Marseille now have a hinterland. It must have an interior territory, and it is here that the Rhône valley takes on its importance."[34] Southeastern France might therefore provide Marseille's "interior territory," or internal empire. After looking outward for millennia, now Marseille had to turn inward. From a "semidesert economy," the southeast could become the ancient city's promised hinterland. The *Grand Delta* association was initially formed out of concern for Marseille following decolonization, but it soon developed its broader, interregional mission for the entire southeast.[35] In particular, Fos, a massive deep-water port and industrial center on the outer suburbs of Marseille that was home to a major oil refinery, might become "l'Europort du Sud."[36] It might help re-anchor Marseille as a center of trade and commerce.[37] Regional development might foster, therefore, the transformation of surrounding rural environments to support the coastal metropole and ensure its continued importance. Rural, provincial France once again became the country's periphery when there was no longer an empire beyond its national borders.

In addition to reviving Marseille, contemporaries also hoped that regional economic development might contribute to the re-equilibration of France as a whole. In particular, the southeast might provide a counterweight to Paris. As Antoine Pinay, chief administrator of the *Grand Delta* association and leading politician of the Fourth and Fifth Republics, put it, "it is fundamental and urgent to rebalance France." Only when there were geographical-economic regroupings of sufficient size "to constitute an indispensable counterweight to the Parisian mass," Pinay warned, would the problem be resolved. The southeast of France was the most promising counterbalance to Paris "because of its economic weight, the dynamism of its actors, and its relative distance from the capital." In fact, it might be the only area in all of France that could carry out this objective. Pinay recommended the creation of new "regional systems" that might restructure the singular relationship between Paris and the periphery. Suggesting the continued power of Gravier's metaphor, such a restructuring would thereby return "vigor and dynamism to what can be called, admittedly with a certain level of exaggeration, but with a powerful force of expression, 'the French desert.'" Enacting interregional equilibrium would therefore provide an effective alternative to the dependency on the Parisian basin.[38]

Fostering urban development was critical to this new geography of power. Not only was it important to "equip" regions, but "urban equipment for counterbalancing metropoles" was of special importance.[39] Helping major regional centers such as Lyon and Marseille was key. Yet fostering regional urban growth threatened to reproduce the "same vice" of the unequal relationship between Paris and the periphery on the regional scale. Provincial centralization should not replace national centralization.[40] "To the contrary," "balanced regions" with diverse economic activities that did not depend on a single sector or a single city were the goal. If their establishment was carried out properly, these regional centers would thus be harmonizing forces rather than destructive ones. Such a balanced approach would have important demographic consequences. While workers might be mobile, appropriate regional development would allow for this mobility "sans dépaysement ou déracinement" ("without deterritorializing or uprooting them").[41] This notable phrase critiqued the ways in which urbanization removed individuals from the land.

Yet it was not only the "equilibrium between Paris and the provinces that remained to be assured." Beyond reviving Marseille and balancing Paris, southeastern France promised "the double equilibrium of national and European development."[42] The creation of the Common Market in 1957 placed national economies in a new light. The title of a piece of promotional literature associated with the 1972 exposition proclaimed: "Le Grand Delta: Un rendez-vous avec l'Europe."[43] Integrating the Rhône corridor "within the framework of the major European axes will make sites in southeastern France as attractive as, and—why not?—even more attractive than the sites of the traditional heavy industry triangle of the Rhine." Just as *le Grand Delta* promised to remake the unequal relations between Paris and the rest of France, "a new equilibrium between northern Europe and the Mediterranean will thereby be established" at the same time.[44]

International pressures thus heightened national concerns over regional disparities. Like most of southern Europe "qui reste en arrière," France lagged behind Germany. References to the industrial and economic powerhouse of the "northern delta" or "heavy industry triangle of the Rhine" explicitly compared these deltas.[45] To make matters worse, northern Italy was becoming a formidable new rival.[46] A number of maps compared the Rhône and Rhine deltas visually, placing their location and relative importance in a European context.[47]

In this European context, France's future was precarious. The country risked becoming to Europe what the southeast was to France. To be competitive in Europe meant improving the overall economic state of the entire nation, but this required accelerating the economic development of "backward" areas of the nation. If not, "it is clear that for us, the French of the south, that there is a danger that we will remain on the margins, and thus be marginal to the economic development of Europe." In short, France had to play catch-up.[48] If it succeeded, it might join powerhouse Germany. If it failed, it would end up a weak player like Spain.[49]

The *Grand Delta* association thus aimed to create economic regions beyond the individual boundaries of the nation-state and on the "European scale," thus situating these areas within a European transnationality. The process of integration would be carried out partly through the construction of regions that might or might not maintain national boundaries: "the realization of the EEC is carried out through the region."[50] At its core, *le Grand Delta* was, then, as much transnational as it was interregional. And the Rhône, "after having served its role as a divider, should now become the great uniter."[51] It could forge links across Europe and help to rebalance the economy of the entire continent.[52] The frequent use of artery metaphors suggested that *le Grand Delta* and the Rhône were critical to the very health of Europe.[53]

Together, the political aim of regionalization and its manifestation in the landscape of the greater Rhône valley aimed to achieve political economic equilibrium. The economies of greater Lyon and Marseille might reach a level of "symbiosis."[54] Yet there were perpetual risks of creating "new economic deserts, and new population deserts." Just as regional capitals might dominate like Paris, big industries might also unsettle local economies. Through diverse activities on different scales, however, it was possible to foster "the harmonious development of the *Grand Delta,* which," one contemporary argued, "seems to be an absolutely indispensable element of the economic riches of France in the Common Market."[55] As part of regional economic development, the Rhône might redeem the region and nation, thus ensuring France a prominent place in an integrated Europe.

After World War II, "Paris et le désert français" posed political and economic problems for France's leaders. In response to the excessive power of Paris and the "backward" state of the provinces, regional economic planning attempted to develop the resources of the French periphery. The regionalization of the Rhône River was born of these perceived tensions between Paris and the provinces. State planners and social scientists hoped that economically, the Rhône might revive its hinterlands and thus contribute to regional and national renewal. With time, challenges to political centralization combined with post-1945 European integration contributed to the creation of regions in France. Meanwhile, economic disparities belied the limits of revolutionary claims of equality and universality. As the history of the river's transformation illustrates, regional economic development established specific institutions and projects like agricultural reconversion to carry out this mission. By the mid-1960s, then, the Rhône was, as one recent scholar has put it, "between nation and region."[56]

In this respatialization of the Rhône and the political economy of France itself, contemporaries viewed cities as both blessings and potential downfalls. Regional renewal depended upon *métropoles d'équilibre* and *métropoles régionales,* counterweights to Paris. Conversely, *métropoles d'équilibre* like Marseille could not thrive alone. They needed rural places. Yet regional cities also posed threats to their hinterlands just as Paris drained the nation. Consequently, during the postwar era, French officials and academics attempted to strike the right balance between national interest and regional demands, between autonomy and dependency, between urban and rural. Substantial government policy therefore aimed to define and manage urban and rural places. Urban and rural environments were thus implicated in fundamental debates over the foundations of postwar French political economy at the very moment when European integration began to call into question the boundaries of the modern nation-state and the very idea of "France."

NOTES

Epigraphs: J.-F. Gravier, *Paris et le désert français* (Paris: Flammarion, 1947), p. 1; Antoine Pinay, "Une alliance d'avenir à l'échelle de l'Europe: Le Grand Delta," *Revue d'action Régionale* (1968): 7.

1. For an extended discussion of this point, see Sara B. Pritchard, "Reconstructing the Rhône: The Cultural Politics of Nature and Nation in Contemporary France," *French Historical Studies* 27, no. 4 (2004): 765–99.

2. Paul Claval, *Histoire de la Géographie française de 1870 à nos jours* (Paris: Nathan, 1998), pp. 223, 444.

3. Quoted in Gravier, *Paris et le désert français,* p. 1.

4. Vivien A. Schmidt, *Democratizing France: The Political and Administrative History of Decentralization* (New York: Cambridge University Press, 1990), pp. 12–15.

5. Ibid., pp. 4, 5.

6. Pierre Deyon, *Paris et ses provinces: Le défi de la décentralisation, 1770–1992* (Paris: Armand Colin, 1992).

7. Ibid.

8. Peter Alexis Gourevitch, *Paris and the Provinces: The Politics of Local Government Reform in France* (Berkeley: University of California Press, 1980).

9. Quoted in Deyon, *Paris et ses provinces,* p. 119.

10. Jean-Michel Hoerner, *Géopolitique des territoires: De l'espace approprié à la suprématie des Etats-nations* (Perpignan: Presses Universitaires de Perpignan, 1996).

11. M. Michel, *L'aménagement régional en France: Du territoire aux territoires* (Paris: Masson, 1994).

12. Hoerner, *Géopolitique des Territoires,* p. 125.

13. Michel, *L'aménagement régional en France,* p. 3.

14. David Barnes, *The Making of a Social Disease: Tuberculosis in Nineteenth-Century France* (Berkeley: University of California Press, 1995); Robert Nye, *Crime, Madness, and Politics in Modern France* (Princeton, N.J.: Princeton University Press, 1984); Ann-Louise Shapiro, *Breaking the Codes: Female Criminality in Fin-de-Siècle Paris* (Stanford, Calif.: Stanford University Press, 1996).

15. Barnes, *The Making of a Social Disease;* Shapiro, *Breaking the Codes.*

16. For a summary of Haussmanization, see Jeremy Popkin, *A History of Modern France* (Englewood Cliffs, N.J.: Prentice-Hall, 1994), pp. 119–20, 131. On Paris sewers, Donald Reid, *Paris Sewers and Sewermen: Realities and Representations* (Cambridge, Mass.: Harvard University Press, 1991).

17. The term "technopolitics" comes from Gabrielle Hecht, *The Radiance of France: Nuclear Power and National Identity after World War II* (Cambridge, Mass.: MIT Press, 1998).

18. For an overview of Vichy's agricultural politics, see Popkin, *A History of Modern France,* p. 235.

19. Jean-Robert Pitte, *Philippe Lamour: Père de l'aménagement du territoire* (Paris: Fayard, 2002), p. 226.

20. Jacques Soustelle, *L'avenir du "Grand Delta" et l'Europe* (Paris: IMP, n.d.), p. 2, Compagnie Nationale du Rhône (CNR), Documentation, AE 0753; Ian B. Thompson, *The Lower Rhône and Marseille* (Oxford: Oxford University Press, 1975), p. 46; "Le Grand Delta: Un rendez-vous avec l'Europe . . . des journées internationales 1972 à l'horizon 1980," *La Vie Française* 1452 bis (1973): 5–7.

21. René Mayer, "Le Rhône, principal axe de transport français," *Delta: Revue d'Action Régionale,* no. 19 (1968): 28–35, CNR, Documentation, AE 0167.

22. "Le Grand Delta," p. 7.

23. Ibid.

24. Pierre Terrin, "Le Grand Delta," *Transports,* no. 147 (1962): 391–94, CNR, Documentation, AE 0167.

25. Thompson, *The Lower Rhône,* p. 46.

26. Pinay, "Une alliance d'avenir," p. 8.

27. "Le Grand Delta," pp. 5, 7, 9–10.

28. Soustelle, *L'avenir du "Grand Delta,"* p. 2.

29. "Le Grand Delta," p. 24.

30. Soustelle, *L'avenir du "Grand Delta,"* p. 6.

31. "Le Grand Delta," pp. 10–11.

32. Soustelle, *L'avenir du "Grand Delta,"* p. 4; Mayer, "Le Rhône, principal axe de transport français," pp. 28–29; Terrin, "Le Grand Delta," pp. 391–92.

33. Terrin, "Le Grand Delta," p. 392; on "la Californie européenne," see Ministère de l'Equipement et du Logement et Ministère des Transports, "Equipement et développement du sillon rhodanien et du Sud-Est français," *Equipement, Logements, Transports* (1969): 9; "Le Grand Delta," pp. 10–11.

34. Soustelle, *L'avenir du "Grand Delta,"* p. 11.

35. "Le Grand Delta," pp. 5, 7.

36. Ministère de l'Equipement, "Equipement et développement du sillon rhodanien," p. 16.

37. Thompson, *The Lower Rhône;* Ministère de l'Equipement, "Equipement et développement du sillon rhodanien," p. 4.

38. Pinay, "Une alliance d'avenir," pp. 7, 9, 12–13; Ministère de l'Equipement, "Equipement et développement du sillon rhodanien," pp. 4, 6.

39. Ministère de l'Equipement, "Equipement et développement du sillon rhodanien," pp. 4, 24.

40. Philippe Lamour, *L'aménagement du territoire: Principes, éléments directeurs, méthodes et moyens* (Paris: Les Editions de l'Epargne, 1964), p. 34.

41. Pinay, "Une alliance d'avenir," pp. 9–12.

42. Ministère de l'Equipement, "Equipement et développement du sillon rhodanien," p. 3.

43. "Le Grand Delta."

44. Ministère de l'Equipement, "Equipement et développement du sillon rhodanien," p. 39.

45. Soustelle, *L'avenir du "Grand Delta,"* p. 11.

46. Thompson, *The Lower Rhône,* p. 46.

47. "Le Grand Delta," pp. 25–26.

48. Soustelle, *L'avenir du "Grand Delta,"* pp. 3–4, 6.

49. Lamour, *L'aménagement du territoire,* pp. 6–7.

50. Pinay, "Une alliance d'avenir," p. 10.

51. Ministère de l'Equipement, "Equipement et développement du sillon rhodanien," p. 6.

52. Mayer, "Le Rhône, principal axe de transport français," p. 33; Pinay, "Une alliance d'avenir," p. 9.

53. See, e.g., the statement of P. Bayard that Rhône projects would improve navigation "in the perspective of the major sea artery between the North Sea and the Mediterranean," "Le vrai visage de l'aménagement de Pierre-Bénite sur le Rhône," *L'Ingénieur,* no. 73 (1967): 25; compare Abel Thomas, *Sillon Rhodanien: Axe-Rhin Méditerranée: Rapport du Commissaire à l'aménagement du territoire* (Paris: R. Lacer, 1960), pp. 155–56.

54. Mayer, "Le Rhône, principal axe de transport français," pp. 34–35.

55. Soustelle, *L'avenir du "Grand Delta,"* pp. 17, 19.

56. Jacques Bethemont, "Le Rhône: Entre nation et région," *Revue de Géographie de Lyon* 72 (1997): 67–75.

Notes on Contributors

Karl Appuhn is Assistant Professor of History at New York University. He won the American Society for Environmental History's 2001 Alice Hamilton Prize for "Inventing Nature: Forests, Forestry, and State Power in Renaissance Venice," published in the *Journal of Modern History.* He has been a fellow at the Columbia Society of Fellows in the Humanities, the American Academy in Rome, and the Institute for Advanced Study.

Joanna L. Dyl is a doctoral candidate in History at Princeton University. Her dissertation is entitled "Urban Disaster: An Environmental History of San Francisco after the 1906 Earthquake."

Andrew C. Isenberg is Associate Professor of History at Temple University. He is the author of *The Destruction of the Bison: An Environmental History, 1750–1920* (2000) and *Mining California: An Ecological History* (2005).

Ari Kelman is an Associate Professor of History at the University of California–Davis. His first book, *A River and Its City: The Nature of Landscape in New Orleans* (2003) received the 2004 Abbott Lowell Cummings Award. He is currently working on a book about the politics of memory surrounding the Sand Creek Massacre.

Matthew Klingle is Assistant Professor of History and Environmental Studies at Bowdoin College. His dissertation, "Urban by Nature: An Environmental History of Seattle, 1880–1970," won the Urban History Association's best dissertation prize in 2001. He has published articles in *History and Theory* and the *Journal of Urban History,* and is currently finishing his book on the environmental history of Seattle.

Emmanuel Kreike is Assistant Professor of History at Princeton University. He is the author of *Re-Creating Eden: Land Use, Environment, and Society in Southern Angola and Northern Namibia* (2004).

Sara B. Pritchard is Assistant Professor of History at Montana State University and has held postdoctoral fellowships at the University of Pennsylvania and the Massachusetts Institute of Technology. Her dissertation,

"Recreating the Rhone: Nature and Technology in France since World War II," was awarded the Rachel Carson Prize by the American Society for Environmental History in 2002.

PETER THORSHEIM is Assistant Professor of History at the University of North Carolina at Charlotte, where he teaches British history, environmental history, and the history of technology. He is the author of *Inventing Pollution: Coal, Smoke, and Culture in Britain since 1800* (2006).

ELLEN STROUD is Assistant Professor of History at Oberlin College and currently a fellow at the Charles Warren Center for Studies in American History at Harvard University, and an American Council of Learned Societies/Andrew W. Mellon Junior Faculty Fellow. She completed her dissertation, "The Return of the Forest: Urbanization and Reforestation in the Northeastern United States," at Columbia University in 2001. She won the American Society for Environmental History's 2000 Alice Hamilton Prize for "Troubled Waters in Ecotopia: Environmental Racism in Portland, Oregon," published in *Radical History Review.*

Index

Page numbers with an *f* indicate figures.

This volume explores the intersection of cities and the natural environment in an array of urban places, including New York, London, New Orleans, Venice, and Seattle, across a broad period from the late Renaissance to the present. The essays investigate the ecological context of revolts-both real and imagined-by urban squatters and slaves; urban epidemics and their cultural and political consequences; the social and economic impact of natural catastrophes upon urban places; and the environmental history of the rise and fall of cities. *The Nature of Cities* brings together the work of scholars employing new methods of research in urban and environmental history. The contributors to the volume, who include Karl Appuhn, Joanna Dyl, Ari Kelman, Matthew Klingle, Emmanuel Kreike, Sara Pritchard, Peter Thorsheim, and Ellen Stroud, represent a new generation of scholars in urban environmental history. Their innovative and interdisciplinary work draws on race, class, consumerism, landscape studies, and culture to address such questions as racial and class conflicts in urban public spaces; the cultural construction and control of public spaces by economic and government powers; and the idealization of cities as apart from nature.

Andrew C. Isenberg is professor of history at Temple University.

Printed and bound by CPI Group (UK) Ltd, Croydon, CR0 4YY

15/09/2026

14962416-0001